FACIAL FITNESS

Revolutionize Your Self–care with Facial Exercises and Holistic Massage Techniques for Neck and Décolletage.

DR. ANDREA BLAKE-GARRETT

In loving memory of Walter H. Garrett, Sr.,
my Vetspouse1.

Thank you for loving me FOREVER!
See you later!

Table of Contents

Introduction

> I can honestly say I love getting older. Then again, I never put my glasses on before looking in the mirror.
>
> **—Cherie Lunghi**

Confidence is key when it comes to growing old gracefully, so why not do what you can to achieve it? Growing older is an inevitable reality of life. There are, of course, several benefits to this maturity, including more wisdom, more financial stability, and an increased independence of thought and action. Yet, it would be naive of me to ignore the fact that there are some aspects of aging that many of us will consider negatives. One of the most prominent occurrences, usually perceived as unfavorable, is skin sagging, especially on the face and neck.

As we move through life, our bones naturally lose density, our muscles weaken, and our skin becomes looser. Because of this, many people in their 40s and 50s will start seeing changes in their appearances, with some people experiencing these signs of aging as early as their 30s. In my book *Live Fit & Free For Life: Exercise for Seniors 60+,* I shared how we can dominate the fears and frustrations associated with aging. Of course, this does not faze everyone, as some people don't worry about how they look as they age, but for many, their perceived attractiveness dramatically affects their self-esteem, and they'd prefer to do something about it.

To some, this desire to look a certain way or slow the effects of aging might come across as superficial, but I believe that if this makes you feel good about yourself and proud of your appearance, there's no harm in giving it a try.

This mindset is what has made the anti-aging industry such a massive success. Millions of people across the globe buy into the idea that we must not look our age and spend a tremendous amount of money on cosmetic surgery, laser treatments, fillers, and creams to achieve what they believe is flawless and youthful skin. Did you know that achieving healthy, glowing, and firm skin on the face, neck, and décolletage doesn't have to be expensive or invasive? In fact, you don't need anything more than the basic information I've collated in this book.

The following chapters include a combination of knowledge and observations from my years of life and research, which I have compiled to produce straightforward, helpful, and cost-effective health and beauty strategies that will help you look and feel your best regardless of gender, background, or age. So, put down the $100 creams and the chemical-laden injections and join me on a far more natural and sustainable journey to a more youthful and healthier-looking you.

Facial Fitness: revolutionize your Self-care with Facial Exercises and Massage Techniques for the Face & Neck and Décolletage is a user-friendly and empowering book; you will discover and learn about:

- The lifestyle choices you make could be aging you faster than you'd like, and how best to avoid these beauty no-nos as we advance.

- The quickest and most effective ways to remove the residue of past bad beauty habits from your face and neck area.

- How to reduce the classic signs of facial aging, such as inflammation and redness, while giving the skin a boost in all it needs to stay healthy and firm.

- Actionable steps for managing and improving specific dermatological flaws, including acne, skin discoloration, physical discomfort, and pain.

- How to level up your facial massage skills and boost its effects with simple tools, oils, and organic lotions.

- The top and most effective massage techniques, yoga moves, and facial workouts proven to improve the quality and tightness of the skin on your face, neck, chin, and décolletage.

- Ancient practices used by different cultures for thousands of years to help them maximize their natural beauty.

Facial massage for beauty has unfortunately developed a bit of a poor reputation on social media or in certain reality TV shows, with some considering it to be fool's gold when it comes to reversing or halting the aging process. However, the truth is that it is common practice in many African and Asian cultures and has been used for centuries to enhance skin elasticity and youthfulness. Furthermore, dermatological professionals and scientists have supported the idea that, when performed regularly, facial massage can give the appearance of lifted and rejuvenated skin regardless of age or lifestyle (Villines, 2022).

As someone who has transformed their skin and body and greatly values mental, emotional, spiritual, and physical health and wellness, practicing facial massage and fitness is exceptionally beneficial. Not only did it reduce my signs of aging, but it also aided detoxification, boosted circulation, and relieved many physical afflictions like headaches and sinus problems. With all of this in mind, I believe we all deserve to know about these practical and surprisingly easy techniques and use them to maximize our goals, not just beautiful or handsome on the outside but beautiful, energized, and confident on the inside too. So, trust the process and join me on your journey to aging gracefully. Show up as your most authentic, marvelous self every day.

Chapter 1:

Fact or Fantasy

> **"** Everything is theoretically impossible until it is done.
>
> **—Robert A. Heinlein "**

There has been a lot of speculation regarding the effectiveness of facial massages when it comes to gaining youthful and glowing skin. Many people believe that they are nothing more than a gimmick and just another way for the beauty and skincare industry to profit from consumer insecurities. However, unlike the many jars filled with empty promises, facial massages work, and the dermatological industry's enormous financial investment has proved this. They have been found to potentially improve the appearance of wrinkles, sagging, and acne, as well as the texture, sinus pressure, and blood flow, all resulting in glowing skin and rejuvenation when practiced regularly and correctly (Cronkleton, 2020).

The evidence in favor of facial massage continues beyond there. It is a practice that has a very long history, originating in African and Asian nations, so it has been able to stand the test of time, suggesting that there is certainly more to it than we think or know.

The History of Facial Massage

African Nations

Throughout the African continent, massage has been used as a form of health, healing, self-love, and meditation for generations for over 4,700 years. In the western part of the African continent, organic shea and cocoa butter are often used to help the hands glide across the faces and bodies of friends, parents, siblings, and babies to demonstrate love for the community.

This ritual has developed over time and became known as *Digui* massage, which is still in use by specific cultural groups from the Ivory Coast, Mali, Nigeria, and Ghana. The *Digui* massage involves long, enveloping, and deep palm-based strokes across the skin. They are designed to knead out tension knots and promote aesthetic and emotional rejuvenation. Natural tools such as rungu stick (made of Eucalyptus or Rubberwood) and calabash were also introduced to provide more profound relief, turning these practices into what is known locally as "happy therapies" with deep spiritual energies.

Digui was traditionally performed on the body, but over the years, it has been adapted to be used on the face to improve mental and dermatological health. Many African cultures now use it for physical and spiritual purposes. Benefits include decreased puffiness, elimination of toxins and surplus fats, stimulation of the lymphatic system, and blood circulation and muscle toning. The result is a smooth complexion and a firmer, natural-looking, youthful face.

China

It is said that the Chinese first used massage therapy nearly 4,000 years ago to promote vitality (Slater, 2020). It was used to spiritually connect with the universe and balance the forces and elements. It was also a type of medicine they believed to reduce stress and provide a space for profound relaxation and healing. From that point, word of its effectiveness and pleasure spread across the globe and seemed to infuse into the practices of other cultures.

As we know, China was one of the first places in the world to develop the notion of massage, with ancient Chinese texts from around 2700 BC describing the therapeutic advantages of massage therapy

(Davids, 2020). Traditional Chinese medicine doctors, martial arts practitioners, Buddhists, and Taoists all believed that touch was an essential component of their spiritual training, and even laypeople would provide and enjoy regular full-body massages for relaxation. This is because massage therapy and other specialized bodywork treatments were believed to allow energy to flow more harmoniously through the body in order to heal itself spontaneously. They used techniques such as acupressure, acupuncture, and tuina while engaging in nutritional changes, herbal medicine, and exercise regimens to maximize the multiple benefits.

In China, face massages, in particular, were developed as far back as the 14th century (Davids, 2020). This type of traditional massage is known as Gua Sha and was widely used in ancient China, initially to heal general illnesses. Still, the technique quickly grew in popularity as it was seen to rejuvenate the skin on the face by removing toxins and giving it a plump, radiant glow.

India

Massage therapy first emerged in India around 3,000 BC or even earlier as a form of sacred healing (Florida Academy, 2019). It was used in Hindu Ayurveda, a type of holistic "life health" medicinal system considered of divine origin and passed down for generations. According to Ayurveda, people become susceptible to illness when they live in disharmony with the environment, so massage is used to restore the body's natural and physical balance so that it can heal.

This idea of using massage to heal remained popular in India, and in the 10th century, Indian head massage was born (Las Santé, 2014).

Popularly known as Champissage, this type of massage involves massaging the scalp with the aim of improving the growth and condition of women's hair. It did this by increasing the flow of oxygenated blood to the scalp, relieving tension in the skin, and boosting the immune system. By the 1970s, the Indian head massage had slowly evolved to include the neck, shoulders, and, yes, the face, and it continues to be a type of massage that heals the skin and re-balances the energy flow in the body for peace of mind and vitality.

Greece

Ancient Greek athletes used massage therapy to keep their bodies in shape before their games. At the time, various medical ailments were also treated using massage techniques when Hippocrates taught his medical colleagues its beneficial effects in aiding the body's natural healing process and recommended using friction to treat physical injuries. It is believed that his knowledge of massage techniques and their benefits came from his time on the African continent.

This rubbing action, in conjunction with aromatic herbs and oils, was eventually used for skin care after realizing the advantages they provided. It was believed that the combination of facial massage and a balanced diet, rest, exercise, fresh air, and music could get the skin of the body and face looking its best. Notice that this sounds very similar to the environment and treatment we use in our spas today, so we still maintain this belief and reap its benefits

Japan

Kobido is an ancient Japanese facial massage that has been about for at least 540 years (The LA Glow, 2021). It came about when two masters of another massage technique, Anma, combined their skills of pressing, stroking, and kneading the body and adapted it for the face to appeal to French clientele. They established 48 new facial techniques, and each was very advanced, taking prodigies many years to master. Over the next 100 years, more than 50 additional techniques were added by the Japanese to this art, and it is now considered so adequate for facial beauty that it has been nicknamed the "Japanese face-lift."

Unlike most of the other ancient massages we have already discussed, Kobido is focused mainly on enhancing beauty and is designed to help sculpt the face, considering one's skin texture, curves, and elasticity—the calming sensation is just a bonus!

As you can see, facial massage is far from a gimmick, and its longevity is a testament to its success in facial rejuvenation and overall skin improvement. After all, a 4,000-year positive track record is pretty impressive!

Misconceptions and Myths

Despite this impressive track record, there are still some misconceptions and myths about facial massages, so before we go any further, I want to debunk them so that you feel even more assured that this is the treatment for you.

Myth 1: Facial Massages Hurt

In the world of natural skin care, pain is a huge no-no. Whether you are engaging in a massage, wash, or cleanse, if it hurts, the likelihood is that you are doing something wrong or are being too aggressive.

With more invasive treatments such as fillers or Botox, some discomfort is to be expected. The techniques included in this book are not invasive. They are all meant to be gentle and beneficial to your emotional, mental, physical, and spiritual health. Always bear this in mind when it comes to gauging the best amount of pressure for you to use during massages. You should also be aware of the products you may want to use and ensure they do not irritate the skin or cause any other adverse reactions. Despite this book being called *Face Fitness*, this is not a "no pain, no gain" situation.

Myth 2: Facial Massages Need to Be Done by a Professional

Professional face massages are great and can be a lovely treat for you to enjoy every now and then. They will have particular expertise and may even have access to specialist products you don't have access to. However, suitable quality treatments can be pretty expensive, especially at the frequency they are required to notice any benefits, so they are unaffordable for most of us. The good news is that self-massage with the right tools and guidance can be just as effective. You may not be able to fall asleep as you perform your own massage, but when it comes to reaping the rewards of youthful and taut skin, you are more than capable of achieving this on your own.

Furthermore, who knows your skin more than you do? You see your face every day, so you understand the way it moves, you know your problem areas, and you know what pressure and products work best for you in the long term. When you go to a professional, as thorough as they may be, there is only so much they can learn from a form and form looking at your skin for a few minutes, so trust your judgment and knowledge about yourself and be confident that you know how to look after the skin you're in.

Myth 3: Facial Massages Cause Breakouts

Some people believe that manipulating the skin on our faces causes breakouts because of the extra oils produced. This belief is a myth! As long as your skin and fingers are clean, and you cleanse your face after a massage, there is no reason why you will be more at risk of acne than you would at any other time.

It is worth bearing in mind that the skin on your face is more delicate than in other areas, especially as you get older. As you age, your hormone levels will also change, so the products or techniques that worked for you in your 20s may not work for you now. With this in mind, start off gently and less frequently to see how your skin reacts and build up from there. If you notice any negative changes in your skin, it could be a sign that you need to step up your facial hygiene or that there is an underlying reason why your skin is reacting that way. If you are worried, always consult a doctor or skin care professional.

Myth 4: Facial Massages Are Just for Women

The media often portrays spa treatments and self-care activities as very feminine. We are used to seeing women in robes attending spas or having quiet nights wearing facial masks, but we rarely see men engaging in such rituals. This is because society has led us to believe that men's skin should be tougher (literally) and that it is more acceptable for men's skin to visibly age. Unfortunately, this is how society has been for many years, but it should not be the case. Self-care has no gender, so it should be enjoyed by all. All skin types can suffer the effects of aging, so there is no reason why men should not take part in facial massage or anything that helps with their confidence and self-esteem.

There are even specific benefits of facial massages and treatments for men; for example, they can rid the skin of excess oil and bacteria. Men are prone to have oilier skin than women due to higher hormone testosterone levels (Gillette, 2019). This oil makes it easier for bacteria to get caught up in the pores, so massaging the face (and cleansing afterward) can eliminate this potentially disruptive bacteria more easily and frequently, leaving room for healthier and clearer-looking skin. Men also tend to sweat more than women, making their faces look clammier, so performing facial massages can be beneficial because they improve circulation to the skin's surface, which tightens pores, thus reducing sweating. Last but not least, for men with beards, face massages can soothe razor burn and visibly calm irritation from itchy hair. Ingrown hairs on the face can cause unsightly bumps, which make the face look more worn and older than it is, so investing in some self-massage is a brilliant way to maintain a smooth and fresh appearance.

Myth 5: I Need Expensive Oils, Creams, and Tools

Remember, expensive does not necessarily mean good quality and high quality does not have to be expensive. When it comes to the substances we put on our faces, they should, of course, be safe, but you should be bold in using natural oils and butters that are found in reasonably priced stores. Some of the best products may be found in our home cupboards because if you can eat them and they are suitable for your insides, the chances are they are just as suitable for you on the outside.

An excellent example of this is coconut oil. Many of us use it for our cooking because it is high in "good fats" and tastes lovely. However, it is also great for our skin because it is rich in vitamin E, which acts as an anti-inflammatory agent and has antibacterial qualities (Jahns, 2022). Moreover, it absorbs very well into the skin and traps moisture, making the face appear more plump, which is an effective way to reduce the appearance of fine lines. Other affordable food products that work well on the face during massages are brown sugar, olive oil, cucumbers, and avocados. So next time you want to reach for that $50 - $100 bottle, go online or take a trip down to the organic market instead.

When it comes to tools for the face, certain items can be more expensive than expected, but these are few and far between. You could get creative and try making your own, but I recommend investing in the natural item to avoid injury or damage and achieve the best results. Remember you will be working with a most sensitive part of your body. Think of these purchases as an investment in your self-esteem, and if you buy a quality rungu stick, calabash, roller or stone, for example, it should last you a lifetime.

Myth 6: Facial Massages Take Too Long

Facial self-massage can take a few minutes to half an hour, depending on how intense you want or need it to be and which areas you'd like to focus on. Some exercises can even be done while watching TV, reading, or at your desk—if you don't mind some intrigued looks—so you shouldn't worry about them taking up too much of your day. That being said, you should never rush through or skip any steps of the massage to shorten the sessions, as each step and its number of repetitions has its benefits, so always try to set enough time aside to complete the entire sequence or workout. Consistency adds excellent value. You are worth it!

If you have a hectic schedule, add some facial time to your day by setting the alarm and making sure it is a priority, as anything that improves your sense of self should be an essential part of life.

Myth 7: Facial Massages Are Miracle Workers

Facial massages and exercises work wonders, but they aren't miracle workers. They still require a holistic sense of self-care, from managing a healthier diet to full body exercise and avoiding harmful habits and thoughts. They can only do so much to give you the appearance of youth, so you'll also need to put in the work in other areas of your life to notice a difference.

You'll also need to commit to doing them regularly, as one session won't have the power to change your skin for the rest of your life. This is because our skin refreshes itself approximately every 28 days, so you should give yourself at least this amount of time to change your entire lifestyle for the better.

I hope I've clarified and removed some of the misconceptions that might have been holding you back from participating in face fitness; you now feel more aware of what is hearsay and factual. Facial massages and exercises should be a positive experience. You should feel rejuvenated after each session. They will excite you about what you'll see in the mirror in the next few weeks or months.

Benefits of Facial Massage

Now that the myths have been addressed, it's time to focus on all the incredible benefits the content of this book is going to bring to your life. You may think I am biased, but trustworthy sources scientifically support all the following benefits and have many success stories to back them up.

- **Fewer wrinkles and slower effects of aging.** As you've purchased this book, this is probably your main reason for giving facial massage and fitness a try, and I am pleased to say that you will find great value here. In 2017, a study was conducted to examine the effectiveness of facial massage in gaining youthful-looking skin. It was found that using nourishing creams and suitable tools helped make wrinkles shallower, the skin tighter, and the skin texture smoother when carried out once a day for at least ten days (Cronkleton, 2020).

- **Reduced acne.** Facial massage techniques that move and manipulate the skin can loosen dead skin cells and decongest the pores, which are both great for reducing the likelihood of getting acne. It is essential, however, to always have clean hands and tools, as rubbing anything dirty on your face can spread bacteria and worsen any acne already present.

- **Glowing skin.** The movement and pressure applied to the skin's surface during a facial massage will increase the blood flow to this area and potentially to the rest of your body. This improved circulation will give you a brighter, more glowing complexion because when blood flows well, it brings oxygen and nutrients to the surface, which prevents skin discoloration. Specific facial massage techniques also encourage drainage, which will eliminate toxins in the lymphatic system. A buildup of toxins in the system can make our skin look dull and puffy, so performing regular massages will be beneficial.

- **Smoother scar tissue.** If you are unfortunate enough to have unwanted facial scarring, performing facial massages can be incredibly beneficial, as the increased blood flow loosens up any hard tissue and can flatten any raised areas. If your scar is still healing, it has been proven that massage can also relieve any unwanted symptoms such as tenderness, itching, and pain, so it is often prescribed for those who have undergone surgery and want to find more comfort during the healing process (Cronkleton, 2020).

- **Improved temporomandibular joint (TMJ) conditions.** The TMJ is the sliding hinge that connects your jawbone to your skull on each side of your face, allowing you to open and close your mouth. Some people develop conditions like arthritis in this joint and the muscles surrounding it, which can cause a lot of pain. Still, discomfort in this area can also be caused by injury, genetics, or even extremely bad habits, such as clenching or grinding the teeth (bruxism).

Research from the Cleveland Clinic has shown that by engaging in trigger point massage on this joint, one can alleviate the tight, inflamed, or painful jaw muscles from these conditions, especially when combined with jaw exercises (Cronkleton, 2020).

- **Reduce puffiness.** If you suffer from a very puffy face in the morning or find that your face feels and looks heavier than it did a few years ago, the good news is that facial massage can reduce the appearance of bloating significantly. Facial puffiness is essentially the presentation of excess fluid retention, so the movement of massage moves and drains this fluid quicker than it would naturally, leaving your skin feeling flatter and less tender. Forget the expensive firming creams. Perform the facial massages I will share daily and achieve better drainage results.

- **A boost in mood.** Not only will facial massage make you look good, but it will also help you to feel good. It has been proven to make us relax, reduce feelings of anxiety, and even improve sleep by relieving muscle tension and activating the sympathetic nervous system, which is responsible for keeping you alert and responsive (Poidevin-Hill, n.d.).

All of these benefits are more than enough reasons to try facial massage, and I'm sure they have excited you to get started. You aren't the only one to be excited by the possibilities of facial massage either, as many celebrities swear by them and are always looking for new techniques and products to keep their faces looking their best. For example, many older celebrities partially owe their glowing and youthful skin to facial massages that use deep massage movements to feel for tension and then sculpt and contour the face by de-stressing the muscle tissue.

Some celebrities are particularly adventurous with their techniques and take facial massage to a new level by opting for treatments like the buccal massage. Jennifer Lopez and the Duchess of Sussex are among those who have tried this unique massage, which involves massaging the cheeks from the inside (Harper, 2023). Yes, inside the mouth. It is said to be a nonsurgical alternative to a face-lift, providing a more sculpted look, but it was initially used to treat patients with Bruxism and Bell's palsy, which both cause discomfort in the jaw. It was developed as a beauty treatment by celebrity "facialist" Nichola Joss less than a year ago, and beauty salons have seen an 85% increase in uptake since launching. This shows that innovation is key, and many people across the globe desire youthful skin, so it is nothing to be ashamed of or secretive about (Harper, 2023).

Things To Consider

Although I won't be talking you through the buccal massage techniques in this book, there are some things to be aware of before starting a facial massage session.

Suppose you have severe acne that is painful and recurring or any other skin condition like eczema or dermatitis. In that case, I recommend speaking to your medical professional before starting. This is because your skin may be very sensitive, and I wouldn't want you to end up damaging or scarring it.

You should also ensure that your nails are relatively short and smooth before engaging in massages. You do not want to injure your eyes. Keep in mind that any sharp edges could snag or scratch the skin, which can be particularly painful in areas like under the eyes or on the lips. Despite these points, facial massage is very safe and can be performed by anyone.

Chapter 2:

Behind the Mask

"Beauty is about enhancing what you have. Let yourself shine through.

—Janelle Monae"

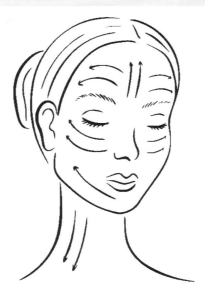

Afamous saying states, "Beauty is only skin deep" but in its literal sense, this isn't true when it comes to facial fitness, massage, and rejuvenation. The attractiveness and youthfulness of a face go much deeper than the skin and has a lot to do with the muscles, fat, and tissues found in the face as well as your lifestyle and what you consume. With this in mind, in this chapter we will be exploring what exactly makes the skin look and feel young and smooth before you even start massaging. We'll be looking at the science behind it and what you need to do behind the scenes to maintain a face you feel proud of.

What Makes a Youthful Face

We may all have different facial structures, skin tones, and thickness in facial hair, but there is a general consensus on what youth looks like. It generally involves having:

- Full firm lips and cheeks

- Firm yet supple skin
- Smooth skin
- Bright eyes
- White and straight teeth
- A clearly defined jawline and firm neckline
- Even toned and hydrated skin

All of these features are associated with youth because, as we age, these things naturally change for a variety of reasons. Our collagen and elastin production slows down, making the skin lose its firmness and elasticity; fat cells start to disappear, which makes our cheeks and jaw begin to sag; hormone changes make our skin less able to retain moisture and new skin cells are generated less often which can make the skin look duller, and pesky gravity generally pulls the skin on our face downward, giving us a less sharp neck and jawline.

As depressing as this may sound, these aging symptoms aren't usually very severe and certainly don't happen overnight. But if you'd like to slow your visible aging process even more, there are certain lifestyle choices you can and should change to help youthful qualities stick around for a little longer.

Maintaining Youth

Have you ever looked at someone and been shocked by their age? Have you ever seen two people of the same age who look entirely different? As long as neither of them has had surgery. As we know invasive, surgical options are no miracle worker. You can tell when someone has gone under the knife. No the younger looking person has a healthier lifestyle. The healthier they are on the inside, the more youthful they'll tend to be on the outside. It would be wise for you to improve your nutrition and increase hydration if you want to increase your chances of achieving and maintaining a healthier and more youthful looking skin.

Avoid Excessive Sunlight Exposure

I firmly believe in the benefits of phototherapy using the sun as the source of light. When exposed to sunlight the skin releases a compound that relieves inflammation. It also helps the body produce Vitamin D which benefits your whole body systems including the skin. I could write an entire book on the importance of Vitamin D to the body. It is essential for maintaining healthier bones, prevents acne and dry skin, decreases inflammation, improves replication process of cells, influence production of collagen, and strengthen skin cells. Whether you have eczema, jaundice, acne, or psoriasis, sunlight is the way to go. It is recommended to limit exposure to 30 minutes a day. Early morning sun is best.

It has been well-documented that excessive unprotected exposure to UV light can cause all sorts of skin issues, from sunburn to cancer; therefore, wearing sunblock is an essential part of daily healthcare (Shah, 2020). If not properly protected, avoiding direct sunlight exposure is good practice if you want to prevent premature aging, as UV radiation can cause wrinkles and dark spots, which both mar the appearance of youthful skin.

However, too much of anything is not good. Extensive exposure to the sun required protection. I recommend choosing natural sunscreens widely available online. They are made with various fruit extracts and oils like Castor oil, Jojoba, Rosehip, Sunflower, etc. You will find out more about these amazing oils in later chapters. Dermatologist Anna Lien-Lun Chien recommends using at least factor 30 Sun Protection Factor (SPF) cream daily or as high as factor 60 if you spend much time outdoors. Many of the more popular brands are full of unhealthy chemicals. It is recommended that you should also shield your skin from the sun using hats or light scarves when necessary and avoid using sunbeds too often. So even if you have beautifully darker skin tones, make applying sun protection and reapplying as recommended a part of your daily routine. Ultimately, the choice is yours.

Quit Smoking

Yes, I said it! Quit smoking. Smoking can kill you fast or slow. Why do you think there is a warning label on tobacco items? We all know that smoking causes damage to our insides and increases our chances of developing cancers, but did you know that it can also age us on the outside? Smoking cigarettes, cigars, whatever can cause topical damage to the skin as it increases the levels of toxins the skin is exposed to. Smoking has also been found to deplete the skin of vitamin C by up to 15%, and this vitamin is responsible for healing. So, if you are a smoker, you might find that scars or wounds on your face take longer to heal than normal (Shah, 2020). As well as this, the act of smoking itself—the constantly pursed lips—can also cause wrinkles known to plastic surgeons as "smoker's lines."

Limit Alcohol Intake

Like smoking, drinking alcohol can seriously affect your skin as it is a substance that causes dehydration and dehydrated skin wrinkles quickly. Drinking alcohol in excess can also make the skin look dull and gray or shiny and red, neither of which is exceptionally youthful or healthy looking. As well as this, regular drinking can cause water retention, making your face look puffy and irritating the blood vessels in the eyes, making them look bloodshot. So try to reduce your intake to no more than two alcoholic drinks per day for men or one drink per day for women (CDC, 2019). Pop star and Billionairess Rihanna told Marie Claire Magazine that whenever she sees her skin deteriorating, she cuts her alcohol consumption down completely and notices a significant difference, so it would be wise to follow in her footsteps.

Avoid an Unhealthy Diet

Eating a lot of fatty food and drinking sugary drinks is a big no-no when it comes to maintaining youthful skin. This is because excess sugar in your bloodstream causes a natural chemical reaction called Glycation, which affects the collagen and elastin in the skin. It makes these proteins weaker, thus reducing the skin's "springy" appearance, which makes signs of aging more apparent.

Some unhealthy fats, like saturated or trans fats found in processed or fried foods, are also known to make the skin very oily, which can cause breakouts. They can also clog the arteries and worsen circulation, which, as we know, can affect the skin's vibrancy. However, it is important to remember that some "good" fat found in avocados, fish, and nuts is needed to keep the skin looking plump and smooth, so choose your meals wisely.

Avoid Dehydration

Dry skin differs from dehydrated skin, and knowing the difference in skincare is essential. Dry skin requires moisture but is not necessarily an indication of dehydration. It can be hereditary and is usually considered a skin type that is quite difficult to change.

Skin dehydration, on the other hand, is when the skin is simply in need of water. It is usually caused by environmental factors such as a change in seasons, or it could be because you've drunk too much caffeine. Fortunately, this can be easily remedied by increasing your water intake, but if you don't, you could find yourself developing red patches, dark circles, and wrinkles.

Get Enough Quality Sleep

Getting enough sleep is probably one of the most underrated anti-aging tools. While you're asleep, your body repairs the skin and lowers stress levels. So if you don't get enough of it, your skin may start to look damaged and your cortisol levels will increase, which is known to increase fat retention. You should therefore aim to get at least seven or eight hours of sleep per night, just like Olivia Wilde. She says she never fully relies on products to make her look "perfect" and instead ensures she has enough sleep every night (Shah, 2020).

Look After Your Gut Health

Numerous studies have found that our gut health can affect our skin (Mirabello, 2019). An unhealthy gut caused by stress, little sleep, and a poor diet can lead to breakouts, psoriasis, dry skin, and eczema. This is because it can prevent your digestive system from absorbing the nutrients you need to maintain healthy skin. An unhealthy gut can also change the way the body metabolizes hormones, detoxifies the blood, and builds the immune system. This is why our skin is often a valuable barometer for what is happening inside us.

Avoid Inflammation

Inflammation can make us look older because it reddens the skin, gives a bloated appearance, and makes the complexion look very patchy. It can happen for many reasons, including immune system problems, allergies, infections, adverse reactions to heat, or photosensitivity. Therefore, boost your immune system by exercising and eating well while treating any underlying allergies, sensitivities, or conditions you might have.

Tracking Your Health

Keeping track of these health and lifestyle improvements is challenging for the best of us. Fortunately, plenty of apps and gadgets do this for you. There are forms of technology that monitor sleep cycles, apps that assess diet and gut health, bottles that help track hydration, and alarms that remind us to do facial massages and exercises on time and for the proper length of time, so be advised to take full advantage of them.

The Healthier Lifestyle

Now that we've addressed the things you might be doing that have adverse effects on your skin let's explore what you should do to achieve the best possible skin.

Introduce Omega-3

Even if you eat a lot of wild caught fish, it is almost impossible to get the recommended amount of Omegas in your diet, so you may want to consider taking supplements daily, as this has been found to improve not only the condition of the skin, but also psychiatric health, eye health, and brain growth (Shah, 2020). Of course, supplements should be taken in conjunction with a healthy diet, so be sure to eat plenty of foods that contain omegas naturally, like mackerel, oysters, flaxseed, walnuts, and soybeans.

Omega-3 is great for our skin because it is a fatty acid that has the power to reduce puffiness. It is an anti-inflammatory agent. It contains a chemical that reduces the production of eicosanoids and cytokines, which are substances linked to inflammation. It also helps support the health of the skin's cell membranes, which promotes hydration and can prevent hyperkeratinization, which is when the hair follicles on the skin's surface become red and raised.

Moisturize Daily

Moisturizing your skin every morning and night is the perfect practice when on the quest to improve the appearance of the skin. Dry skin is easily irritated, so deodorant soaps and products that contain alcohol or fragrance can irritate your dry, sensitive skin. This is because dry skin can make once-plump skin cells become dry and shriveled, leading to premature lines and wrinkles. By moisturizing, especially after a bath or shower, you'll be trapping water in your skin, which temporarily hydrates it and helps fill any small lines and creases. Adding gentle, fragrance-free skin care products is highly recommended. Opting for natural oils such as organic hexane-free castor or avocado oil would be best. It would be best if you were consistent in maximizing your internal skin health, as surface moisturization is often temporary.

Eat a Balanced Diet

Our diet plays a huge role in our skin condition because, as the famous saying goes, "you are what you eat." The body needs very specific nutrients to be able to, not only function properly, but also to look its best and most of these nutrients can be absorbed through a fresh, varied, and balanced diet.

According to the Federation of American Scientists, a balanced diet for the typical adult consists of "two and a half cups of vegetables, two cups of fruit, six ounces of grains, three cups of dairy, five and a half ounces of protein, and 27 grams of oil" every day (White et al., 2021).

Hydrate More

When you think you've drunk enough water for the day, drink some more. Mix it up with those hydrating fruits, juices or juice blends that include cantaloupe, cucumber, strawberries, tomatoes, watermelon, etc. The average person's daily water intake isn't high enough, so it is likely that your body could do with another few glasses right now. Water might not taste of much and drinking more may make you urinate more than usual, but these cons certainly do not outweigh the pros, so I recommend that you add a slice of lemon or cucumber to your glass or bottle and challenge yourself to drink at least eight glasses every day.

Aside from keeping the skin plump and hydrated, drinking enough natural juices and water also helps maintain a good pH balance in your skin. The ideal pH level for the surface of skin is between 4.7 and 6, which means it should be slightly acidic (White et al., 2021). This level is ideal because that is good for keeping lipids and moisture in, while blocking germs, toxins, bacteria, and pollution out.

If you find that your skin is very dry and sensitive, it could mean that your pH levels are too high (alkaline) or if it is very red and inflamed, it could mean that it is too acidic. Fortunately, keeping hydrated with liquids at or near a neutral pH of seven has the power to balance out your skin's levels, whatever the case may be, and leave it smooth and resilient.

Take Probiotics

The gut is full of live bacteria and yeasts that help it and the digestive system work at their best. Sometimes, this "good" bacteria get depleted because of a poor diet or infection, and we need some help to top the levels back up to what is considered healthy. This is where probiotics step in to save the day! They are essentially consumable versions of these bacteria and yeast.

It might sound strange for me to advise you to consume bacteria, but we all need certain types of it to break down our food properly.

Probiotics can come in tablet or liquid form and are usually easy to find in your local drug or convenience store. Still, you can also gain a healthy amount of good bacteria from everyday food items. For example, unpasteurized sauerkraut, certain natural yogurts with live cultures, kimchi, and kombucha are good sources of lactic acid bacteria and yeast.

Sleep Deeply

After lying in bed for a few hours or napping for short periods over the course of the day, you may feel relaxed and refreshed temporarily, but sleeping every night is very important, not only for your skin but also for your overall health.

Deep sleep, also known as slow-wave sleep, occurs during the third stage of non-rapid eye movement (NREM) sleep when our brain waves are at their slowest frequency and highest amplitude. This typically happens about an hour after initially falling asleep. It is when your heart and breathing rates are at their slowest and your muscles are fully relaxed, so napping for a few minutes probably won't get you to this point.

But why is *deep* sleep so important? Well, during this time, your body releases growth hormones, and it's when memory and cognitive skills are improved. It's also when your muscles, bones, and tissue, including the skin, are built and repaired. Without enough deep sleep, your body won't be able to regulate glucose metabolism very well either, which can affect the skin's bounce, leaving it looking flat and sunken. So, try not to pull "all-nighters" too often, even if you have a deadline to hit.

Exercise

In my book, *Live Fit & Free For Life: Exercise For Seniors 60+*, I outline the health benefits of consistent exercise. The information shared in this book is true whether you are 30, 40, 50, or older. Getting the oxygenated blood pumping around the body through cardiovascular exercise is an excellent way to keep your skin looking bright and youthful. Regular exercise will also help you to lose body fat, which will generally make you look slimmer and more youthful, but it can also positively affect the look of your face in particular. This is because when we age, the fat pads in our lower face—pockets of stubborn fat that sit under the skin—tend to become fuller and rounder, which can cause this area to sag and alter the overall shape of your face. Exercising and losing excess fat can help stop this from happening too obviously. You should join a fitness team, exercise at home, join a gym, run with friends, or enjoy swimming at your local pool.

I devoted an entire chapter to the benefits of Resistance/Strength training in *Live Fit & Free For Life: Exercise For Seniors 60+*. Resistance or Strength training involves the use of weights or body weight to build muscle— should also be added to your exercise schedule because, after the age of 30, the body's muscle mass starts to decrease by up to 5% per decade (Perkins, 2021). This is called sarcopenia and is usually caused by hormone changes such as testosterone, human growth hormone, and insulin. Therefore, resistance or strength training is necessary to keep your body toned and counterbalance this natural effect of aging. Many might not know that your facial muscles work the same way. For this reason, muscular exercises are incorporated in the upcoming chapter that discusses face fitness techniques to help you sculpt your face.

Massage Your Face

Last but not least, of course, we have a facial massage. It is a natural way to even out the complexion, tone the facial muscles, improve circulation, and much more. Introducing it into your routine will feel great and, over time, will leave you looking vibrant and youthful. But before diving in and poking and prodding your face haphazardly, it would be wise to learn exactly what parts of your face should be massaged and why so that you can achieve the results you desire.

Understanding the Face and Neck Muscles

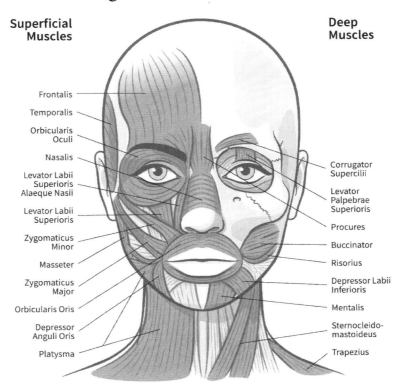

Whenever we laugh, cry, cringe, or chew, the muscles in our faces contract and relax to create an array of intricate movements. In fact, human beings are capable of making over 100,000 expressions, each portraying a different emotion using just under 20 different flat skeletal muscles in the face and a few more across the rest of the head region (CBC, 2019). The seven most prominent muscles, however, are:

- Frontalis is on the front of the forehead and is used to raise eyebrows.
- Temporalis on each side of the head near the temples are used to aid chewing.
- Orbicularis oculi, which goes around the eyes and controls blinking and squinting.
- Zygomaticus major and minor, which go from the corners of the mouth to the top of the cheekbone and help you smile.
- Orbicularis oris, which circles the mouth and helps you to pucker up for a kiss, pout, and whistle.
- Buccinator at the cheeks also helps with whistling, chewing, and blowing.
- Masseter, which is toward the back of the jaw and aids with chewing too.

In the neck, there are 20 muscles that also have an influence on facial movement and structure, and they are grouped by location: anterior (front), lateral (sides), and posterior (back).

- **Anterior neck muscles.** One of the main muscles in this region is the platysma, which runs from below the collarbone to below the mouth. You can feel it contract if you downturn your mouth or grimace. The other main muscle group is the sternocleidomastoid, which goes from the middle of the collarbone to just under each ear. It is used to rotate and flex the neck.

- **Lateral neck muscles.** The leading muscle group in this area is the scalenes, which are three pairs of muscles that are found on the sides of the neck and control the lateral flexion of the neck. This is when you move your ear to your shoulder.

- **Posterior neck muscles.** There are quite a lot of important muscles in this region, the largest being the trapezius. This is a considerable superficial muscle that resembles a trapezoid running from the back of the skull all the way to the lower spine and across the top of your shoulders. It allows you to extend the neck and even helps with shoulder and upper limb movement. The splenius capitis is a deeper muscle that supports the head when upright and runs from the base of the skull to the bottom of the neck. The splenius cervicis is another deep muscle that also aids the support of the head while in motion. Finally, the levator scapulae, which go from the neck to the shoulder blades, help move the neck side to side and the shoulder blades up and down.

I don't expect you to remember all of these technical names, but it is helpful to know which muscles control what and where they are located so that you can identify your "problem" areas to target when you start massaging. For example, if you want to improve the tension of the skin and muscles around your chin, you now know that it may be worth paying attention to not only the top of the neck under your chin but also the cheeks and the back of the neck, as there are muscles that move and support the chin in these places as well.

Dos and Don'ts

Despite the muscles in our face and neck being able to produce so many intricate movements and supporting the heaviest and most vital part of our bodies, they are relatively sensitive and delicate when compared to the leg or arm muscles, for example. This means that extra care is needed when manipulating and touching them, and there are things you should and shouldn't do to avoid injury, pain, or complications. There are also some general rules when it comes to facial massage and fitness, which are essential to remember for the best results.

Dos

- **Massage upward.** Massaging in an upward motion on the face helps to counter the effects of gravity. Also, rather than going back and forth in a rubbing motion, always stop at the top of the stroke and start again from the original position. This motion should also be used whenever you are applying lotion or skin care products.

- **Start at the décolletage.** The décolletage is the upper chest area, below your chin and above your cleavage. It is a very delicate area, and it is prone to damage because of its exposure to the sun and the fact that many of us neglect it in our skincare regimens. You should always start here and move up toward the face when massaging the neck, as it will pull the skin up against gravity, elongate the neck, and avoid sagging.

- **Move from the inside of the face out.** This motion helps open out the face, making you look and feel alert. So always start from the inner corners of the eyes, bridge of the nose, or inner eyebrows and pull out toward your hairline, ears, or chin.

- **Use a range of motions.** There are different motions used in facial massage, which we will go into more detail in Chapter 4, and it is helpful to mix these up throughout your session as they each have different benefits. Circular motions are suitable for general relaxation and improved circulation; lifting motions help with sagging, and tapping will help increase blood flow to the specific area.

- **Be consistent.** Unfortunately, one massage and stretch session per week won't cut it when trying to achieve youthful skin, so aiming for at least 10 minutes each day is essential to reap maximum benefits.

- **Know your skin type.** Before you add any products to your routine, knowing whether you have dry, oily, or combination skin is vital. This will help you choose the best products for you, as you will be using them daily and don't want to worsen any underlying issues or cause irritation. If your skin is oily, you can still use natural oils on your face. Your face should not be dried out. I will provide detailed information about these face oils in upcoming chapters. It is not an all or nothing situation.

- **Work both sides of the face.** Nobody wants a lop-sided face, so be sure to massage and exercise both sides equally so that you aren't left with taut, youthful skin and dull, blemished skin on the other.

- **Improve your posture.** Hunching your shoulders at a desk or looking over a cell phone for long periods can be detrimental to your posture. Bad posture can then make the skin around your neck and décolletage wrinkle and crease prematurely. So, working on keeping your shoulders back, neck straight, and chin parallel to the floor will help prevent this from developing into a problem.

Don'ts

- **Don't use a lot of pressure around the eyes.** The skin around your eyes is probably the most sensitive on the body. Your eyes are also very precious, so it is wise to move around this delicate area gently and softly. A little pressure goes a long way in this location.

- **Don't press too hard.** Even in areas away from your eyes, you shouldn't be pressing hard enough to see any indentations. Pressing too hard could cause skin trauma, leaving long-lasting scarring or bruising, which is the opposite of what we want to achieve.

- **Don't forget to use oil or cream.** Not using oils or creams during your session can cause a lot of friction and will pull and stretch the skin in ways we don't want. So, if you don't have any oils, it would be best to wait until you do. The oils will allow your hands or tools to glide smoothly along the skin and avoid scratching or bruising along the way by reducing the amount of friction.

- **Don't push. Always pull.** Pushing the skin in any direction can cause a wrinkling and rippling effect, which we want to avoid. So no matter what part of the body you are working on, always use a pulling motion by shifting your hand position. It is a subtle difference, but it will have lasting effects when done regularly.

- **Don't rush.** Take your time performing facial massage because we only have one face and any mistakes that leave a long-lasting mark. These massages and exercises are meant to be pleasurable and beneficial, so try to see it as some well-earned you-time.

All the suggestions in this chapter will help make the process of attaining a youthful glow much smoother, so do your best to follow them all while using the upcoming massage and exercise techniques.

Chapter 3:

Massage Must-Haves

> **"**
>
> Massage is not just a luxury. It's a way of a healthier, happier life.
>
> **–Unknown**
>
> **"**

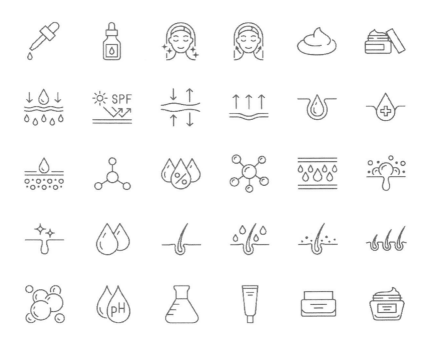

Although you can perform facial massage without any products, some items are believed to help you achieve quicker, more sustained, and more holistic results. Some essential tools are also required to perform precise techniques like cupping or gua sha, so additional purchases are necessary if you'd like to try these. These products should not cost more than $40 or $50. These items don't have to be expensive, nor must they be the newest gadgets on the market or from a well-known brand, but if you are going to invest in face fitness for life, then quality is critical.

Creams and Lotions

There are hundreds, if not thousands, of different beauty products on the shelves, each claiming to tighten, radiate, smoothen, plump, and rejuvenate the skin. But which ones should we choose? It mainly depends on your skin type and your desires. For example, if you have very dry skin and want to improve the plumpness of your face, you should use hydrating products that target deep layers so that your skin can hold onto moisture for as long as possible throughout the day. If you have very oily skin, however, you may want to avoid heavy creams or items that contain alcohol, menthol, mint, or aromatic oils, as these can stimulate the oil production glands and make your oily skin worse. Instead, opt for lighter, more effective cleansing organic products and keep a clean oil-sapping pad.

Let me state for the record that organic creams and lotions are highly recommended by this author. Our skin is extremely susceptible to the absorption of whatever it comes in contact with. The consistent use of unnatural toxic chemicals and or contaminants found in many facial creams and lotions can contribute to serious health problems like cancer, hormone disruption, birth defects, and reproductive harm. Organic creams, lotions and oils are best even if you have "oily skin".

According to dermatologist Dr. Anita Sturnham, when you plan to apply your products should also determine which ones you use. Why? Because our skin has its own 24-hour clock. It is known as a circadian rhythm, which means that its anatomical and physiological needs change throughout the day (Davidson, 2023). During the daytime, the skin is more sensitive. It, therefore, needs protection from external factors like pollution and extensive exposure to sunlight, so SPF creams and those that add protective layers should be used. In the evening, however, the skin starts repairing itself, so products with nourishing ingredients like vitamins E and C would be more helpful. Again, there are natural and vegan sunscreens widely available on the cosmetic market.

Not only are the type of products you use essential for maintaining healthy skin but also the order in which you apply them to your face. Different products have different absorption rates, and using them in the "wrong" order could weaken their effects (Davidson, 2023). The general rule is to apply the most effective and organic product with the thinnest consistency first and end with the cream or lotion that is the thickest. With this in mind, Cosmopolitan magazine recommends following a morning routine like this:

1. **Cleanser.** After washing your face, start the day by applying a light cleanser to remove any remnants of oils or sleep left on the skin. It should be gentle, non-abrasive, and hydrating and leave the skin ready to absorb a toner. Many effective natural oil-free cleansers on the market contain a mixture of natural plant extracts, naturally known as hydrators, including plant-based hyaluronic acid, that won't remove valuable oils from the skin.

2. **Toner.** Water-based toners help rebalance the skin's pH levels. Toners are liquid moisturizers designed to tone your skin—tighten pores, and reduce inflammation—by providing it with goodness like oxygen, hydrogen, and essential vitamins and acids. Natural toners such as rosewater lemon juice or even watermelon juice, are best.

3. **Eye cream.** It's not recommended to use the same cream on the rest of your face around your eyes. This is because the skin in the eye area is much thinner and more sensitive, requiring a lighter yet more hydrating product that helps boost collagen levels. Creams and serums rich in hyaluronic acid and peptides are great for this, as they help structure the cells. Many doctors recommend applying these creams in thin layers throughout the day, along with other serums that are designed to penetrate the skin deeply. Those that contain vitamin C, vitamin B5 (panthenol), and ferulic acid are particularly good.

4. **Moisturizer.** Once you've hydrated the eye area, you should moisturize the rest of the face with non-pore-clogging creams or lotions containing ingredients like safflower, apricot kernel, and squalene. Remember to always apply your moisturizers in an upward or circular motion to help your skin retain its fight against gravity! There are a variety of oil serums for sale. These are packed with natural essential oils that are known to have anti-aging, anti-inflammatory, and anti-bacterial properties.

5. **SPF.** We've already discussed that you should always apply SPF to protect your skin when exposed to the sun for extensive periods of time.

If you wear makeup at the end of each day, it is imperative to remove it thoroughly with face wash and warm water. A light exfoliant can also be used every few days. You should then gently wipe your face with a cotton pad to get anything stubborn out of the skin—on the last wipe, your pad should be clean. Sticking to this routine will help prevent breakouts and any discoloration over time.

You should then repeat Steps 1 and 2 from your morning routine and apply product rich in Vitamin A. This vitamin is the go-to substance for fighting signs of aging at a deep cellular level. It helps reduce fine lines and wrinkles. How? It promotes collagen and elastin production while reducing pore congestion by regulating sebum production and reducing inflammation—no wonder it's the holy grail of anti-aging! For this reason, it is good at aiding the healing process that happens when you are asleep. Just remember, a little goes a long way.

After applying oil rich in Vitamin A, a good nighttime moisturizer is essential. It should be thicker than your daytime product to ensure that all the great products and healing energy remains in the skin during your eight hours of sleep. If your moisturizer contains Vitamin A that is even better.

Of course, not everyone can afford such an array of products, or you may prefer to keep your face routine minimal. If this is the case for you, stick to just a few natural organic products with a proven track record for achieving your desired outcome. You can still fight aging as long as the products are pure and safe for the skin. You'll also be in good company, with celebrities embracing natural alternatives like rosehip oil, Jojoba oil, castor oil, almond seed oil, and even their own mix of yogurt, honey, and turmeric for their skincare regimens.

I highly recommend avoiding any creams, lotions, oil mixtures that contain BHT or Butylated hydroxytoluene. This chemical is being linked to a number of health issues including prevention of blood clotting and tumor growth worldwide. Foods and cosmetic products containing BHT have been banned in many countries. The United States is not one of those countries. Be informed!

Natural Alternatives

If you are someone who prefers to use organic products or enjoy making your own herbal concoctions to improve your well-being, there are natural alternatives to synthetic products that have similar if not better qualities when applied to the skin. For example, hibiscus, pomegranate, and baobab seed oil contain peptides, so when crushed and added to face masks, they can nourish the skin greatly (Nakin Skincare, 2020).

Tip #1: Use of spices like turmeric and fruits to create an organic rejuvenating face pack. Simply mix a pinch of turmeric powder with a little curd or mash ripe papaya fruit into a rough pulp and apply this to the face for about 5-10 minutes.

Tip #2: Aloe vera gel straight from the plant as a cooling, anti-inflammatory moisturizer or garlic and sandalwood oil as protection against acne. In fact, there are many oils that add great value to your facial appearance and state of mind.

Oils

Natural oils have been used for massage for thousands of years, as they reduce friction, allowing the hands to glide across the skin without causing too much friction. Many natural oils have additional properties that are also nutritious for the skin and can be a healthier alternative to mass-produced chemical filled creams and lotions. Some of these oils and their benefits are listed below.

Coconut Oil

Almost every household has a tub of organic coconut oil somewhere, whether used for the face, body or cooking. This is because it is full of vitamin E, vitamin K, and fatty acids that are good for both our insides and outsides. It also has antifungal and antibacterial properties when used on the face, and a little goes a long way in the protection of the skin from external toxins like smoke or pollution.

A word of caution, however, is that when used on a face that is already oily or prone to acne, coconut oil can provoke breakouts, so it should be used sparingly. However, it can be blended with other oils for a more positive outcome. Great facial oils are:

- Rosemary oil is known under eye puffiness & dark circles. Rosemary is known for targeting under eye puffiness & dark circles.

- Tea Tree known to tighten pores, hydrates skin for softer, and fights daily acne causing bacteria. One of my favorite oils to use. Read the ingredients to ensure that there is no BHT mixed in the oil.

A mixture of Coconut, Tea Tree, Rosemary, Vit. E oils daily is excellent for all skin types.

Sunflower Seed Oil

Another oil, rich in vitamin E, is sunflower seed oil. It is also easily absorbed into the skin and has been found to protect against some forms of eczema (Ludwig, 2020). If applied too liberally, it can leave a sticky residue, so be mindful of how much you use if you choose to use it as a moisturizer. It is excellent, however, for massage. An added benefit is the oil can be easily removed after each session. For the face, Sunflower oil offers maximum hydration while leaving pores unclogged.

Organic Extra Virgin Olive Oil

Olive oil, preferably extra-virgin olive oil, contains vitamins A, D, E, and K, which we know are necessary for healthy skin production. "liquid gold," as the Phoenicians called it, was used by the ancient Greeks used it to moisturize the skin and shine to the hair. It has anti-aging, hydrating, strengthening, toning, healing, and anti-oxidizing properties. The oil can be used as a nonaggressive makeup remover. Olive oil's heavy consistency also gives it the potential to be an excellent moisturizer. Not all oils are alike. Some companies mix other oils in their bottle

African Shea Butter

This thick, whipped butter melts to a rich, smooth oil at body temperature. It is perfect for use as a daily moisturizer, especially during the winter months. It is derived from the nuts of the West African shea tree, which are roasted and then pounded into a paste that solidifies into the butter we see on the shelves and in various hair and skincare products. Shea butter oil is better than liquid gold.

The butter or oil truly nourishes the skin, containing over 50% Oleic Acid and the highest amounts of Stearic Acid and Vitamin E. It is known to condition, tone, and soothe the skin, leaving it moisturized for several hours without reapplication. It absorbs quickly into the skin when applied, leaving a silky, smooth, non-greasy finish. Shea butter has also been related to promoting the production of collagen and slowing down the breakdown of cells in the skin, making it a premier anti-aging oil. Use daily to maximize your facial skincare.

Jojoba Oil

From Africa, we move to South America. Here we'll find high-quality jojoba oil. This oil has so many unique qualities that benefit the face immensely. It is anti-inflammatory and has wound-healing effects while being a fantastic moisturizer, antioxidant, and soother. It doesn't block the pores, and because of its vitamin E content, it is just as good as coconut oil for healing scars, reducing wrinkles, and clearing the skin of bacteria.

Almond Oil

Of course, if you are allergic to nuts, this oil is not for you. But for everyone else, it is a good vitamin E, zinc, proteins, and potassium source. It is lighter than olive oil or shea butter, so it is preferred by most when looking for a face oil. These qualities make it an oil to try if you have dark circles under your eyes or even stretch marks on the neck and chest. It can even be used as a gentle makeup remover that doesn't leave a residue.

Castor Oil

Castor oil can serve as a natural ingredient to your beauty regimen – its hydrating and anti-inflammatory properties make it perfect for skin ailments and a secret weapon for hair and nail health! Castor oil has so many benefits that two or more additional chapters would be needed to introduce it appropriately.

Now, you may be wondering what gives castor oil (Organic Cold-Pressed Hexane Free versions) its remarkable properties. The answer lies in a superhero molecule called Ricinoleic acid. This unique bendy structure is responsible for Castor oil's one-of-a-kind qualities. It affects how it interacts with other molecules and how it behaves in various scenarios. Think of it as a key that fits into every lock. In this case, it's the locks of our body's systems that benefit from its presence.

- Anti-inflammatory ally: Inflammation—the root cause of many health woes—meets its match in Ricinoleic acid. Castor oil has a knack for soothing inflammation. It's like a calming balm for irritated tissues, which is why castor oil's topical applications have been revered for their anti-inflammatory effects for centuries.

- Hydration hero: This unique structure of Ricinoleic acid makes it hydrophilic. This means it is incredibly attracted to water molecules. This translates to enhanced moisture retention, making castor oil a go-to remedy for dry skin and hair. It's like a natural moisture magnet. It works well in treating many conditions, such as eczema.

- Gut guardian: Ricinoleic acid doesn't just stop at skin deep. When ingested, it can also lend a helping hand to our digestive system. Its mild laxative effect can promote healthy bowel movements and ease occasional discomfort. And here's the thing: it does this without disrupting the delicate balance of our gut.

- Millions of pregnant women swear by castor oil's magical prowess in helping them have a smooth and safe delivery.

- Serves as an acne reducer and wrinkle reducer.

Grapeseed Oil

Grapeseed oil is antioxidant, antimicrobial, and anti-inflammatory, so if you suffer from inflamed, discolored, or uneven skin, this could be an excellent oil to introduce into your face care and massage routine. Yet again, it's an oil packed with vitamin E and essential fatty acids.

Argan Oil

This Moroccan favorite, Argan oil, can be applied directly to the skin to reduce inflammation due to injury or infection. Due to its anti-aging ability, it is a popular ingredient in hair and skin care products.

Rosehip Oil

Not to be confused with rose oil, rosehip oil is pressed from the fruit and seeds of the rose plant. It provides the skin with nourishing vitamins and essential fatty acids that keep it looking hydrated and plump. It also contains phenols that have antiviral, antibacterial, and antifungal properties (Ludwig, 2020). Africans, Mayans, and Native Americans have used this ancient oil. Ancient people used to cure a weak stomach, muscle cramps, cough, and colds. When a 1983 research study at the University of Santiago revealed the Rosehip seed oil skin regenerative properties, it became widely used in the skincare industry. Want to smooth wrinkles and minimize scars? Use Rosehip oil.

Aromatherapy and Essential Oils

Some oils not only feel good on the skin but also make us feel good when we inhale their fragrance, and these are known as aromatherapy oils. Aromatherapy is the practice of inhaling or applying certain oils topically to benefit from their scents. These oils are usually essential oil—extracted from plants—and are highly concentrated, giving us positive sensations when we smell them. Use in small amounts when applying to your skin.

Aromatherapy works because when the scent molecules from the essential oils are inhaled, they travel from the olfactory nerves to the brain and impact the amygdala, which is the emotional center. They then trigger a response that makes us feel calm, joyful, or invigorated and rejuvenated. Some of the best oils for these positive reactions are:

- **Frankincense oil** is a precious biblical oil used for grounding and relaxation.

- **Geranium oil** has floral tones that can mentally transport you to a beautiful flower garden. It can also act as an astringent, giving the skin a more toned appearance. Still, it should always be mixed with a base oil before applying it directly to the face.

- **Lavender oil** is probably the most popular essential oil. It is known for its relaxing properties and floral scent that promotes sleep and pain relief.

- **Coriander oil** is less prevailing, with few people recognizing it as an oil used for aromatherapy. However, it has a sweet, warm scent that is soothing and can even promote good digestion (natural Body, n.d.).

- **Bergamot oil** has been used for hundreds of years to reduce feelings of stress and soothe skin. It has a spicy, citrusy aroma, helping to improve your mood and leave you feeling rejuvenated and refreshed.

Using aromatherapy with these essential oils will help you dominate the time spent massaging your face while reducing any stress that may have been disrupting your sleep or making you frown more than usual. Each of these things can contribute to an aging look, so aromatherapy may be the help you need to notice better results from your massages.

Warning: It is important to note that you should not use essential oils neat on the skin, no matter how great they smell. This is because they are highly concentrated and considered irritants, causing the skin to burn, itch, or become inflamed. So, always mix them with any other oils mentioned in this section to dilute their concentration. Just a little is all you need.

Choosing Your Oils

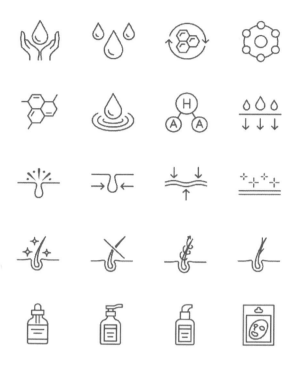

According to the Center of Excellence, the oils you use on your face should not just be chosen for their general qualities or fragrance but also for how they work with your particular skin type.

They suggest the following base oils for each type:

- **Normal skin:** Sweet almond oil or olive oil

- **Dry/more mature skin:** Avocado oil

- **Oily skin:** Jojoba oil

- **Combination skin:** Grapeseed oil

- **Sensitive skin:** Apricot kernel oil

- **ALL skin types:** Castor oil

A few drops of the following essential oils can also be added:

- **Normal skin:** Lavender, ylang-ylang, or jasmine

- **Dry/more mature skin:** Rose, neroli, or sandalwood

- **Oily skin:** Geranium, cedarwood, or lavender

- **Combination skin:** Neroli, lavender, or geranium

- **Sensitive skin:** Rose, lavender, or chamomile

The oils mentioned above can be used alone or blended together, depending on the results needed. Rose Hip Seed, Argan, Sunflower, Vitamin E, are excellent oils to use. Some benefits are:

- aid in wrinkle prevention/ reducing

- tighten sagging skin

- fades dark spots by removing dead skin cells

- brighten & hydrates aging skin

- heals scars

- gives skin a firmer, fresher look by helping to remove toxins and water build-up skin.

Of course, if you have any known sensitivities or allergies, always avoid any irritating oils. If you are unsure, perform a patch test behind the ear or on the wrist. Add a small drop on the area and leave it there for at least 24 hours without washing it off. If you do not react, you are good to go!

Supplements

Nothing beats working on our beauty from the inside out, so taking supplements is a good choice to make, while applying creams or oils topically. They should be taken alongside a healthy and balanced diet and, no matter how desperate you are to see improvements in your skin, you should not exceed the recommended amounts. Unfortunately, that could do more harm than good. I do not recommend solid pill form. It is estimated that only 20% of nutrients, taken in pill form, are absorbed by the body for use. Chewable tablets are best but liquids are better.

Collagen

Collagen is a protein found in the body and is important in the formation and structure of our bones, muscles, tendons, digestive system, blood vessels, and skin. It provides elasticity to the skin, helps wounds heal, and protects the nervous system.

There are, in fact, several different types of collagens, but the most common types are hydrolyzed, undenatured, and gelatin, which are all derived from animal sources. Most come in capsule form, but some collagen supplements are powdered and can easily be added to cakes, smoothies, or even teas and coffees as it is highly soluble and virtually tasteless. Whether liquid, solid, animal, or plant, collagen should be taken as directed.

For improved skin and hair health, it is recommended we take 2.5–10 grams of collagen peptides orally every day for 8–12 weeks (Jacob, 2021).

Vitamins C, E, D, and K

If you struggle to get the recommended amount of vitamins into your system via your diet, taking supplements is a helpful way to top them up. All vitamins are needed to maintain a healthy body, but the main types required for healthy skin, in particular, are vitamins C, E, D, and K. It is important to consume vitamins with a high absorbency rate. You do not want to be flushing your money down the drain.

Vitamin C is found abundantly in citrus fruits such as oranges and lemons, as well as in popular food sources like broccoli, spinach, and strawberries, so deficiency of this vitamin is quite rare. However, if you do find yourself falling short, the general recommendation is to take supplements to bring you up to 1,000 mg per day. This will help protect the cells of your skin and maintain the antioxidant qualities of the outer and middle layers (Bowman, 2020). Vitamin C also has a role in collagen production, so taking these two supplements alongside each other will be helpful.

Vitamin E is another antioxidant found in the skin, but its main function is to protect us against sun damage. It is usually produced through sebum, which is the oil released through the pores, but if you fail to produce enough of it and have particularly dry skin, most healthcare professionals will recommend taking a regular supplement.

The only way humans naturally produce vitamin D is through sunlight exposure and to get a healthy amount into our system, we would need to be in direct sunlight for approximately 15 to 30 minutes per day, every day. Unfortunately, many of us live and work in environments that make this near impossible, especially in winter months. We should also be very mindful of excessive exposure to the sun, so, for these reasons, supplements are beneficial.

In terms of dosage, approximately 600 IU of vitamin D per day is recommended to help create healthy skin cells, but this highly depends on your natural skin tone and how much sun exposure you tend to get, so always double-check your recommended supplementary dosage with your healthcare provider.

Finally, vitamin K is needed to heal the skin, as it supports the body's blood clotting process. It also reduces scars, dark patches, and stubborn circles under our eyes, so it is a vitamin often found in eye creams or products that treat skin conditions. The University of Florida suggests that adults should have between 90 and 120 ug per day, so if you fail to reach this by eating food like kale, spinach, lettuce, and beans, you may want to consider taking supplements (Bowman, 2020).

Fish Oils (Omega 3s)

Fish oils such as cod liver oil contain fatty acids that improve the appearance and health of the skin. They play an important role in skin function and can benefit those with skin conditions such as atopic dermatitis, psoriasis, and skin ulcers. Therefore, taking supplements to ensure that you have approximately 1,000 mg in your system per day will work wonders for your skin (Kubala, 2022).

Multivitamins

Taking multivitamins daily can be helpful for those who struggle to eat a varied diet. They are a quick way to get all you need in one dose, and it was found that most people do benefit from them after approximately 3 months of use. For example, a 2019 study found that significant improvement in skin dullness, dryness, and pigmentation can be achieved, especially if one has underlying deficiencies or insufficiencies (Kubala, 2022). Some items, however, can contain a lot of bulking agents that aren't so healthy and can reduce the absorption of the vitamins themselves, so try to choose good quality products.

Face Fitness Tools and Accessories

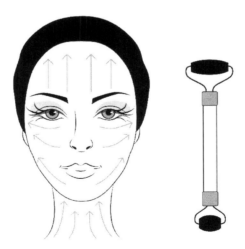

As nifty as our fingers may be, sometimes they can't perform the job required for an effective massage, and we need a bit of help in the form of massage tools like the Calabash and Rungu stick mentioned earlier in this book. These tools, natural or man-made, also take the strain off our fingers and palms and offer new textures that benefit the skin even more.

Facial Cups

Facial cups are small, usually silicone cups that create suction when applied to the skin. They are available in a range of sizes for different areas of the face and are used to briefly separate the layers of facial tissue in order to bring nutrients and blood to them quickly.

These interesting tools are relatively inexpensive, and with their rise in popularity after being associated with various media celebrities and influencers, they are pretty easy to find online. They provide a unique sensation and are used in the facial cupping technique I will be guiding you through in the next chapter.

Rollers and Stones

A face roller is a handy gadget usually made from wood, jade, or rose quartz. Most look like mini-paint rollers, but others may have two balls at the end of a handle. They are designed to roll along the skin and provide a firm, even pressure along a wide surface, which could be hard to achieve with just the fingers. Because of their material, these rollers also offer a cooling sensation which can be great for reducing puffiness, so try cooling yours in the fridge or in an ice bath for additional benefits.

The stone typically used for facial massage is known as the gua sha stone, and it is often flat and shaped like a traditional artist's paint palette. This, too, is usually made from gemstones such as rose quartz, jade, or amethyst, and when performing the gua sha massage technique, it is used to gently scrape against the skin to improve circulation.

Dry Brush

A dry brush in the world of massage is pretty self-explanatory. It is a firm-bristled brush that is used to brush the skin while it is dry. It shouldn't be so firm that it irritates the skin, but stiff enough to invigorate.

Dry brushes are often used in circulation or drainage massage, as they increase blood flow to the surface of the skin and help move toxins around and out of the body via the lymphatic system—more on this later! Dry brushing also stimulates the nervous system in ways that leave you feeling energized.

There are also, of course, plenty of electrical devices that help you exfoliate and massage the skin, but throughout this book, we will be focusing on manual techniques. Manual tools offer a more tailored experience and tend to be less harsh on the face.

Massage tools can make a world of difference in the effects of facial massage, but unfortunately, they aren't much use if you don't know how to use them properly. So, in the next chapter, I will be guiding you through the different techniques and how best to execute them.

Cooling Pads and Masks

If you suffer with under eye or general facial puffiness, cooling pads and masks are designed to reduce this by restricting the vessels under the skin. This restriction stops excess fluid from building up in these areas, which reduces the appearance of inflammation.

These pads and masks are usually filled with gel that stays cool for extended periods of time and are placed under the eyes (or over the entire face) for approximately three to five minutes. So, store them in your fridge overnight or freezer for a few minutes to get the best results.

A more natural method calls for the use of cucumber slices. Cucumber is 96% water. Known for its hydrating and anti-inflammatory properties of cucumbers reduce swelling, moisturize the skin, and stimulate new cell growth.

DIY Tip#1: Grab two cucumber slices from the refrigerator, place on clean dry skin and relax for a fifteen minutes.

DIY Tip #2: Blend ½ - 1 cup of cucumber and 2-3 tablespoons of water until a smooth paste. Be sure to add a tablespoon of fresh Aloe Vera flesh or Aloe Vera gel into the blender. Place the paste on your face for 15 minutes. Wash off with warm water. Follow with the moisturizing oil of your choice.

Facial Gadgets

As well as these well-known tools, there are some other unusual yet innovative gadgets that have filtered into the beauty industry. There are jaw exercises you can use with a small hollow silicone ball to simulate biting, giving your jaw a workout for approximately 5-10 times a day. You can strengthen and lift the facial muscles, creating a defined jawline and tighter cheeks. However, results vary and once training stops, the appearance of the face was found to return to its original shape very rapidly (Johnson, 2020). Remember, consistency is key!

Another gadget for face fitness is the "mouth exerciser", which is essentially a spring-loaded plastic rod. It fits across your mouth, with each end in the corners, and you are required to squeeze and release the rod using only your mouth muscles. It claims to tighten the skin and specifically reduce fine lines around the mouth.

There are also neck pumps or rollers, mouth-powered flapping devices, and "lip exercisers". Unfortunately, most of these fail to have any lasting results and end up being very expensive home decor! Thankfully, there are things you can do without these novelty items that have been proven to make a difference sculpting and toning your facial muscles and skin long-term.

Chapter 4:

Top Massage Techniques

> **"**
> Touch the body. Heal the
> mind. Calm the spirit.
>
> **—Anonymous**
> **"**

If you have ever visited a spa and enjoyed a body massage. There are several different types, each with its benefits and techniques. You'll usually find deep tissue, Swedish, sports, shiatsu, and aromatherapy massages on offer. The same applies to facial massages, so in this chapter, we will discuss the different variations so that you can decide which are most suitable for your needs and preferences.

Types of Facial Massage

Swedish

This popular body massage can also be extended to the head and face. It is known as the base of all other massage types and involves performing long gliding strokes along the skin and kneading and tapping on the soft tissue. Swedish massage is believed to have been founded by Henrik Ling and was introduced to the United States in the late 1850s as "The Swedish Movement Cure" (Swedish Massage—The Complete Guide, 2018). Due to its relatively light touch, its primary purpose is to provide overall relaxation and ease emotional or mental stress, so if you find that you have a lot of tension in your face that is causing you discomfort, irritation, or low mood, for example, this would be a suitable type of massage to try.

Lymphatic Drainage

Lymphatic drainage is the process of eliminating toxins from the body via the lymphatic system. If you are fit and healthy, the body can usually complete this process by itself; however, if you have undergone surgery, had certain medical conditions, or experienced some bodily damage, your body might struggle and need a helping hand through massage.

This type of massage involves manipulating the face in ways that help activate the lymphatic detoxification process.

Reflexology

Reflexology is applying localized pressure to specific points on the body—known as meridian points—to affect one's mind, body, and spirit positively. Most of us are familiar with this being performed on the feet, but it can also be performed on the face, with similar results, as there are meridian points all over the body. On the face, they are located on the forehead, at the temples, between the eyebrows, on and by the sides of the nose, under the eyes, on the upper and lower cheeks, above the upper lip, on the chin, and on the jawline.

According to Chinese medicine, each of these points are linked to other, less accessible parts of the body, so applying pressure in these places can heal internal ailments efficiently while improving our functionality holistically (Wallersteiner, 2020). For example, pressing on the temple or chin is believed to improve the functioning of the kidneys while restoring emotional health and energetic balance.

Two main methods of massage inspired facial reflexology. The first is the Dien Chan, which is a method created by Dr. Bùi Quốc Châu. It is used to stimulate energy channels and has roots in traditional Vietnamese and Chinese medicinal systems. Dien Chan is based on the idea that energy flows through specific points of the head, which can then be harnessed and redirected around the body for our benefit. The second influential method is the Sorensensistem Method, created by Lone Sorenson and uses Eastern and South American techniques for a similar outcome.

It is a prevalent massage concept and has even been known to be prescribed by medical professionals alongside traditional treatment for anxiety, stress, depression, and extreme fatigue (Wallersteiner, 2020).

Shiatsu

Shiatsu is a type of massage often put under the umbrella of reflexology, as it involves putting pressure on certain points with the fingertips. In fact, the word shiatsu is Japanese and means "finger pressure." Applying pressure to these points will enhance blood flow to the entire body and help your muscles relax, relieving general stress and anxiety. This will help you to sleep better, and, as we know, good quality sleep is beneficial to the skin. So, if you lose a lot of sleep or become very anxious about day-to-day life and are concerned about the effects this is having on your skin, shiatsu could be a technique worth trying.

Acupressure

Facial acupressure is a type of massage that also uses the fingers, palms, and knuckles to apply pressure to our meridian points. It is also considered a type of reflexology. Unlike shiatsu, however, it is usually used to treat specific areas of concern. It can help with anything from headaches to congestion and can reduce tension in the jawline, depending on where you press. It also increases cutaneous blood flow—the supply of blood to the skin—and improves lymphatic drainage, all of which can help your skin look more radiant.

According to Health Wellness, the best meridian points to apply pressure to for glowing, youthful skin on the face are the "third eye," "four white," "windscreen," and "facial beauty" points (DeSantis, 2020). The third eye meridian is the center point between your eyebrows, and pressing here for 30 to 60 seconds stimulates the pituitary gland, which is said to help enhance the appearance of frown lines. The "four white" points are near the top of your cheekbones, about a finger-width below the eye socket, and massaging here is said to alleviate blemishes. For radiance, the "windscreen" points behind the earlobes should be pressed, and for an overall glow, massage the facial beauty points at the sides of your nose.

Not much pressure is required to reap the benefits of acupressure, so don't press too heavily, especially around the eyes, as you may experience redness or irritation.

Gua Sha

Gua Sha is an ancient Chinese healing massage that involves scraping the skin with a small, flat stone. It is believed to improve circulation and lymphatic drainage, reduce inflammation, and release tension in the face and neck, so it is excellent for the reduction of puffiness, fine lines, and dark circles.

"Gua" means scrape, and "sha" means tiny, flat red and purple spots in Chinese, which refers to the redness that usually appears after receiving this massage. This redness is nothing to worry about, as it is simply a sign that the scraping is invigorating the blood flow and bringing oxygenated blood to the surface, which is precisely what we want to happen. Just remember that the scraping shouldn't hurt, and you should just look a little flushed afterward rather than bruised and sore! The redness is also temporary, so you should return to your standard skin color within a few hours.

Remedial

Remedial face massages are all about sculpting the face by triggering the muscles around it, giving a taut yet supple appearance. The strokes start at the décolletage and move upward along the neck before arriving at the face, melting away stress and puffiness along the way. The primary goal is eliminating excess pressure, but systematic detoxification is also a huge benefit. So, remedial massage is a wise choice if you want to eliminate toxins or suffer from congestion or temporomandibular conditions.

Sinus Massage

The sinuses are small, air-filled spaces in your skull that help filter and moisten the air you breathe. They also affect the sound of your voice and provide structural support for your face and eyes. There are four different types of sinuses in the face: the ethmoidal, maxillary, sphenoidal, and frontal, and unfortunately, they are all prone to infection. During an infection, they become blocked with mucus, which can be very uncomfortable and leave you looking, feeling very puffy and tired, and sounding pretty bad. Fortunately, sinus massages have the power to improve this almost instantly.

There are two types of sinus massage to combat this congestion. The first is a general massage, which addresses all sinuses via the forehead, and the second is massages that are geared toward each specific sinus. Still, the idea behind both is to apply pressure to each region and help the mucus drain out. This might sound pretty gross, but the relief you'll feel afterward will be immense and very much worth it. So, if you are recovering from a cold and have a heavy feeling in your face or notice that your voice is sounding groggy or restricted, sinus massage should be able to help you out.

Massage Techniques

Various techniques can be used within these different types of massage, each providing a different sensation and benefit to the skin. Some methods were initially used on the body, which, of course, has larger surfaces to work with, but over time, they have been adapted for the face. Therefore, the following techniques are some of the best for the face and neck areas and can be learned quickly, even by those of us who have no background in massage or have never invested in self-care before.

Cupping

You might have seen videos or images of people with large, round glass cups on their backs that are sucking skin up into them. This is undoubtedly an unusual sensation and definitely a strange sight to behold, but it is a technique that has many benefits for the skin.

Cupping is a Chinese and Middle Eastern technique traditionally executed by heating the inside of glass cups with fire and then applying them to the skin. As the cups cool, suction is created, which pulls the skin and bodily fluids to the area, saturating the tissue with fresh blood. This drawing of oxygenated blood and white blood cells to the surface promotes vessel formation and removes toxins, which makes the skin heal and regenerate faster. Over time, this invigoration will give the skin a rich glow and can noticeably improve firmness.

When cupping is performed on the face, smaller and softer cups are used without heat, so the suction is gentle but enough to make a difference in your complexion. You may even notice some redness afterward, but this is entirely normal, and your complexion should return to its usual color shortly after.

1. Start with a clean and dry face.

2. Gently massage your face with the pads of your fingertips to release any superficial tension and warm the skin's surface up. Ensure you are gentle around the eyes and pay attention to the forehead, cheeks, and chin.

3. If you have some light facial oils (highly recommended), apply these now sparingly and evenly across the face. This will help decrease your risk of bruising as you move the cups around.

4. Apply a cup to your chin or near your mouth by squeezing it and allow the suction created to hold it in place for a few seconds.

5. With your face relaxed, slowly drag the cup, still attached to your skin, upward to a new area near the upper jaw or earlobe. Repeat this action on both sides of the face several times,

remembering to remove the cup at the top of the action by gently releasing the suction. Always start again at the chin.

6. Repeat this suction and dragging action from the center of the forehead out to the temples, and from the sides of the nose out to the ears.

7. For smiley areas around the eyes or lips, swap the cup for a smaller one and repeat the action, always moving in the recommended directions.

8. Continue cupping until you have covered all desired areas. This should take approximately five to eight minutes to complete thoroughly.

9. Once complete, wash and cleanse your face to reopen your pores and then pat dry.

10. It would be wise to continue with your beauty or skincare routine soon after this session, as facial cupping is said to improve product absorption, meaning you'll get more out of your face products. BAM!

Unfortunately, if you have a thick beard, cupping the chin and jaw area won't work, as you need a smooth surface to execute the action correctly, but feel free to perform it in regions with minimal facial hair.

Digital or Knuckle Kneading

This technique uses your fingers or knuckles to press into the face in a kneading motion, much like when kneading bread. It requires a little more pressure than most of the other techniques I will discuss in this section, so it is best performed on more extensive and robust facial areas such as the forehead, cheeks, and jawline.

The force created during this technique breaks down and realigns the collagen fibers in the skin, making it lie flat and taught so; this is useful if you tend to frown a lot or suffer from facial tension and pain.

1. Form a fist with your hands and use your knuckles to firmly press into the skin.

2. While maintaining pressure, gently rock your knuckles back and forth as you glide them across the skin in an upward motion.

3. For more sensitive areas, such as the temples or around the mouth, your fingers can be used instead to manipulate the muscles in a similar kneading action.

Rolling

Skin rolling is a massage technique used to release and clear obstructions such as muscular knots and adhesions within the soft tissues. This makes the skin appear smoother as it will be able to flow over the body without any lumps and bumps, so it is effective for softening scars and making the face feel more supple.

1. Use your thumb and fingers to pinch the skin and pull it away from the deeper tissue.

2. While maintaining your grip, gently move the skin around.

3. Continue squeezing and moving motion in any areas of the face you feel are holding tension.

Effleurage

Effleurage is a technique that is used a lot in Swedish massage. It is a continuous stroking motion performed with the fingers in a slow, rhythmic manner, as though you are brushing crumbs off your face. Only light pressure is required to make the experience very relaxing. It is excellent for increasing blood circulation, and because of its gentle and slow movements, it can also stimulate the production of feel-good hormones, such as oxytocin and endorphins.

1. Using the pads and lengths of your fingers, gently brush along the surface of your face in a light sweeping motion.

2. Move around your entire face using this same motion until you have addressed all areas.

3. Remember always to go upward and outward to combat the forces of gravity.

Tapping

Tapping is another very relaxing technique when used on the face. Also known as the percussion technique, it involves tapping the face rapidly with the fingertips as if you were playing a piano. These taps can reach deep into the soft tissue, increasing blood flow and nerve stimulation. As there is no pulling involved, this technique is relatively free, and you can start and end wherever you like, as long as you cover your entire face.

Vibrations

Vibrations can stimulate soft tissues and nerves while relieving muscular tension and stress. Most people will rely on electronic devices to achieve this technique as it can be pretty tricky to perform on your face by hand, but you can certainly give it a try using the lengths and pads of your fingers.

1. Firmly place your fingers flat on a surface of your face that tends to feel quite tight or even numb.

2. While keeping your fingers in place, vigorously vibrate or shake the area for a few seconds.

3. Repeat this shaking motion as you move around the face.

Jacquet Pinching

The Jacquet pinching massage technique was developed in the 1930s by a doctor of the same name (L'Oréal Paris, n.d.). Dr. Jacquet used it to treat war injuries, but it has since developed into a beauty treatment. It uses small and rapid kneading and pinching movements across the entire face to increase circulation and "wake up" the underlying nerves and tissues. It also warms up the facial muscles, making them appear more toned, firm, and plump.

This particular technique should be performed "dry" (without oil) so that your fingers don't slip when pinching the skin at speed. Much like tapping, it can also be started anywhere on the face as long as you move around evenly.

1. Use your thumb and index fingers to perform quick pinching movements with your fingertips. Ensure that your nails are short to prevent any injuries or scratches.

2. Move around the face (avoiding the eyes), continuing this pinching as you go.

Each of these techniques can be used in isolation or alongside each other during one massage session. Just think about what you want to achieve and choose them accordingly.

Later in the book, I will also guide you through how to incorporate them into a routine, so try practicing them now, see how they feel, and get your technique where it needs to be for massage success.

Massage Success Stories

Facial massages can really make a difference to your appearance, as writer Erika Veurink told Byrdie after trying daily massages for just a week (Veurink, 2022). She found a reduction in puffiness and noticed that her face looked and felt more defined, even when taking into consideration her bone structure and the angles she was looking at herself. She said that her "eyes appeared more vibrant and less puffy," and she "looked better rested overall, with [her] jawline a little sharper than normal," so the results speak for themselves, and I'm keen to know what wonders it works for you!

Chapter 5:

Drainage and Circulation

> Massage is not just a luxury,
> it is a way to a happier
> healthier life.
>
> —Anon

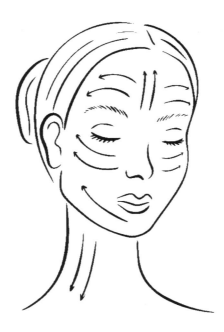

Now that you know the theory, it's time to put this knowledge into practice and learn about the methods and techniques that will allow you to start this exciting anti-aging and rejuvenating process. Clean hands and tools are essential for all the messages outlined in the following few chapters, so always maintain good hygiene to avoid unwanted effects.

Lymph Drainage Massage

As we know, the lymphatic system is one of the body's natural waste removal systems, but occasionally, it doesn't work very efficiently without some assistance. Some visible signs that your lymphatic drainage process is in need of help are puffiness around the face as the lymph fluid builds up, dullness around the eyes as the increase in waste products takes effect, and congestion in the sinuses as the body finds it more challenging to fight the toxins and infections.

Fortunately, lymphatic drainage massage is very effective in treating these symptoms by removing blockages and preventing the lymph fluid from exiting the body. In fact, it is so effective that those with congestive heart failure, a history of blood clots or stroke, a current infection, or liver and kidney problems should not attempt it without speaking to a medical professional first, as it may conflict with their current treatment.

The aim is to use strokes that move toward the lymph nodes in the face, where the toxins and excess fluid can escape. They are located under the outer corners of the jaw, in the neck, and by the ear.

Recommended oil(s): A light serum mixed with citrus essential oils can add significant value. Citrus oils are detoxifying, so they are a great addition to drainage massages. Oils like, Argan, Coconut, Grapeseed Sweet almond, Organic Jojoba, etc. Essentials oils like Lemongrass, grapefruit, orange, peppermint, and ginger add great value.

Optional tool(s): Gua sha wood, stone or a jade roller.

Drainage Tips

- Mainly use gentle effleurage or digital/knuckle kneading techniques to help move the fluid without squashing the lymph nodes.

- Work in upward and outward motions—don't pull down—and massage in small circular motions.

- Be gentle around your eyes. As much as you want to reduce puffiness in this area, it is very sensitive. So take your time to avoid any bruising or poking.

- Keep your skin well-lubricated with oils or creams, apart from when performing the dry brushing technique. Again use essentials oils sparingly. A few drops will do.

- Use your fingertips rather than your palms for more controlled pressure. For deeper pressure, use your knuckles. Be careful of your eyes if you have long nails.

- If using a gua sha tool, only perform a localized back-and-forth "scraping" motion on fine lines and areas of hyperpigmentation. Doing this around the entire face can cause excessive redness and even discomfort.

Massage 1 – Long Strokes on the Face

1. Warm up the skin with light effleurage strokes all over the face.

2. Start at your chin with flat fingers and slowly glide your hands along your jawline towards your ear with light but firmly maintained pressure. Stop below your earlobes and hold this pressure at the ears for a few seconds.

3. Repeat this motion five to ten times, always starting at the chin.

4. Next, put your fingers on the sides of your nose and apply a small amount of pressure. Hold here for a few seconds, then

glide the fingers out and upward toward your ears, taking particular care around your eyes. Use a figure eight pattern if using one hand to massage.

5. Repeat this motion five – ten times, always starting beside your nose.

6. Apply a small amount of pressure on the inner corners of your brows and hold for a few seconds. Move in an outward direction along the brow and toward the temples. Be sure to reduce the pressure when you arrive at the temples because they are relatively delicate. Too much pressure here can cause headaches or disrupt a major artery beneath (Health & Well-being, n.d.).

7. Repeat the steps 8 and 9 five to ten times. Take deep cleansing breaths regularly.

Massage 2 – Circular Motions

1. Place your index and middle fingers underneath your ears and apply gentle pressure. While maintaining this pressure, make tiny circles for approximately 10 seconds. Another option is to, instead of making full circles, make small J shapes going back down, then looping up toward the ear.

2. Now, place these fingers on both sides of your neck—where your arteries are—and apply very light pressure. Maintain pressure and make the same circular or looping motion ten times.

3. Next, place your index and middle fingers on both sides at the base of your neck and apply pressure. Maintain pressure and make the same circular or looping motion ten times.

4. Now, place all your fingers in the soft part, just above your collarbone, and apply gentle pressure as you repeat the circular or looping motion another ten times. Repeat these pressurized circles on the chin, under the corners of your mouth, and at the top corners of your jaw.

5. Now repeat this entire sequence (steps 1 to 8). Take deep slow cleansing breaths regularly.

These circular motions can also be performed on the face at the following locations:

1. at the bottom of the eye socket. Be careful of your eyes, and don't apply too much pressure.

2. at your cheekbone, below the outer corner of the eye.

3. in front of your ears.

4. above your eyebrows.

5. at the temples, very gently.

Immediately after completing these drainage massages, you may need to swallow more than usual or feel some mucus in your throat. This might feel unpleasant, but the good news is that it's a sign that you have achieved drainage! Remember to inhale deep in through your nose and exhale out through your mouth. Breathing exercises are extremely valuable here.

Massage 3 – Gua Sha Stone or Roller

1. Warm up the skin with a few effleurage strokes across the entire face and apply a light oil coating. I highly recommend cold-pressed hexane-free Castor oil, organic Jojoba oil, or cold-pressed Rose Hip seed oil.

2. Place the flattest side of your gua sha stone or roller on your chin, and then sweep the tool along your jawline and up to your right ear. Hold here for a few seconds.

3. Now, position the tool behind the earlobe and then drag or roll the tool down the neck while maintaining pressure. This is the only place a downward motion should be used, as you are trying to move fluid from the jaw to the lymph node in the neck.

4. Repeat the sequence—steps 2 to 3—three times, and then repeat on the left side of the face and neck.

Using these tools can be a little harsher on the skin than our fingers, so this type of massage should be completed at most three times weekly.

Massage 4 – Dry Brushing

Dry brushing is best performed before showering or bathing to wash off any excess oils or dead skin cells that have been disturbed. It should be performed on dry skin, but if uncomfortable, you can add a light oil to the brush, not your face. There are some rules for using dry brushes, as they can cause irritation if misused.

- If you have particularly sensitive skin, use a softer brush or even a dry washcloth instead. If this still causes swelling, excessive redness, or inflammation, stop immediately; unfortunately, this tool is not for you!

- Never perform dry brushing over warts, moles, or raised bumps. They may get caught on the brush and cause damage to the skin.

- Never perform dry brushing on broken or damaged skin, which includes cuts, lesions, scrapes, burns, or bruises. This can cause infection and damage the skin further.

- Purchase a brush that is exclusively for the face. Dry brushing can be performed on the entire body, but using a separate tool is best to avoid cross-contamination. The skin on the face is far more sensitive to bacteria than other areas, so you could end up with breakouts if you share tools.

You're ready to begin once you know and are comfortable with all these.

1. Stimulate the lymph nodes near both sides of your collarbone using your brush to perform small circles in the area for a few seconds. Pressure should be light, and the movement should be relatively quick.

2. Place the brush behind the right earlobe and perform small strokes down the neck until you get to the collarbone. Repeat this five times.

3. Next, place the brush back behind your right earlobe and perform small circles for a few seconds. Although you are performing rotations, think about moving the fluid down toward the collar to get the best "wicking" motion.

4. Now, starting with the brush at your chin, make small strokes up and along the jawline toward your right ear.

5. Continue this brushing motion of small strokes down the neck again and toward the collarbone.

6. Repeat steps 4 and 5 five times.

7. Place the brush just above the lip and create small strokes as you move across the face and toward the right ear. Repeat this five times.

8. Next, place the brush on the bridge of your nose and make long sweeping strokes from the side of the nose to the right ear, following the eye socket. Repeat five times, being careful of the eyes.

9. Finally, place the brush in the center of the forehead and perform small strokes out to the right temple. Repeat five times.

10. Repeat this entire sequence on the left side of the face and neck for balance.

Improved Circulation Massage

Having good circulation is imperative for feeling and looking healthy. Every inch of the body needs a blood supply, so the body's largest organ—the skin—is no exception. Its essential nutrients and oxygen are delivered via the blood, and this particular system is known as cutaneous circulation.

Cutaneous circulation happens through an intricate network of blood vessels and capillaries that exclusively feed the skin with oxygen-rich blood while transporting carbon dioxide and waste products away. Without this constant blood circulation, toxins will build up, and you may end up with dull skin and frequent breakouts.

Fortunately, the following massages will promote blood flow and improve the efficiency of this system in no time.

Recommended oil(s): Almond seed, Castor, Clary Sage, Peppermint (mixed with a base oil). These oils are invigorating and will stimulate blood flow wherever they are applied. My routine requires the use of Organic Cold-Pressed Hexane-free Castor oil. It naturally increases blood flow and improves circulation.

Optional tool(s): Gua sha stone or a roller. If you have a texture roller, this can be even better for stimulation.

Circulation Tips

- Mainly use effleurage, tapping, kneading, and pinching techniques.

- Lubricate the skin with oils or creams before you start.

- Use your fingertips for more controlled, localized pressure, but the lengths of the fingers are better for larger surfaces like the forehead or cheeks.

- Slightly deeper pressure can be used around your cheeks and forehead, but be gentle around your eyes.

- If the knuckles provide a pressure that is too firm for you, feel free to use your fingers instead for massage.

Massage 1 – Knuckle Lifts

1. Sit on a chair before a table or flat surface and rest your elbows on it. Hold your hands up, palms facing you. Your hands should be located on either side of your face. Your elbows should remain on the table for this exercise.

2. Make fists with your hands, then gently press your knuckles into the hollows of your cheeks.

3. Lean forward and rest your cheeks against your knuckles to increase the pressure slightly. Allow your face to relax.

4. Hold this pressure against your cheeks for about a minute.

5. Repeat as desired.

Massage 2 – Rapid Motions

1. Use your fingertips to tap or drum on your forehead.

2. Steadily continue this technique as you move your fingers all over your face for a minute.

3. Next, lightly pinch the skin rapidly and continue this all over your face for another minute.

Massage 3 – Rolling

Keep your roller at room temperature for improved circulation, or slightly warm the surface with your hands. This will keep the blood vessels under the skin dilated, which will help the blood flow freely as you massage. No roller! No Problem! Use your hands with your favorite oil.

1. Place the roller on your chin and slowly roll toward your right ear. Repeat this motion ten times, starting at the chin each time.

2. Next, place the roller by the side of your nose and slowly roll out toward your right ear. Repeat this motion ten times, starting at the nose each time.

3. Next, place the roller in the middle of the forehead and slowly roll it toward your right temple. Repeat this motion ten times, starting at the center of the forehead each time.

4. Now, carefully place the roller by the inner corner of the right eye. Slowly roll out toward your right ear, making a curve under the eye to avoid sensitive areas.

5. Finally, carry out steps 1–8 on the left side of the face.

Massage 4 – Acupressure

As we know, acupressure relies on applying pressure on the meridian point in the face.

For improved circulation and glowing skin, as well as overall well-being, the best points to use are:

- **LI20:** The nasolabial grooves are the grooves on the sides of your nostrils.

- **GV26:** The groove between your lips and nose.

- **Yintang:** Between your eyebrows and where the bridge of your nose meets your forehead. This is also commonly known as the "third eye."

- **Taiyang:** The temples. These are delicate areas where the face slightly dips in at the sides of your forehead.

- **SJ21:** Just in front of your ear by the tragus. The cartilage piece is located on the inside of ear, right in front of the ear canal opening.

- **SJ17:** Just behind the ear lobe at the top of the jaw.

Use your fingertips to apply medium pressure at these meridian points for 10 seconds.

Other points around the body can promote better circulation on the face and beyond, based on the principle of reflexology. Use acupressure in these areas to fascinatingly "wake up" the face weekly.

These are:

- **LI4:** The webbed part of the hand between the thumb and the index finger.

- **LU9:** The bottom inner corner of the palm. As well as circulation, this point is known to improve facial paralysis.

- **Ball of the foot:** Yes, your foot. This area has links with the sinuses and can help drain any excess mucus.

Overall Glowing Skin

Suppose you are fortunate not to have any particular issues with puffiness or circulation and want to maintain glowing skin for as long as possible. In that case, the following massage is for you. It will give you a natural glow and leave you looking and feeling refreshed and ready to tackle the day.

1. **Forehead:** Place all your fingertips just above your eyebrows and apply slight pressure. Slowly push the skin up toward your hairline. Hold for 1-2 seconds, and repeat this motion five times, starting at the eyebrows each time. You can close your eyes.

2. **Eyebrows:** Gently pinch your eyebrows at the inner edge using your thumb and index finger. Move your fingers along the brows to the outer edge, squeezing as you go, and repeat five times.

3. **Eyes:** With your eyes closed, place the tips of your middle and index fingers on your temples and gently massage this area for 10 seconds. Glide your fingers along the bottom of the eye socket toward your nose. Then, slide them up to your eyebrows and across the brow back out to your temple. Never lose contact with your skin; repeat this oval shape around your eyes five times.

4. **Sides of the face:** Starting at the temples again, use the same fingers to make short brushes out toward your hairline. Continue this motion down the sides of your face toward your jaw and repeat consistently for 30 seconds.

5. **Jawline:** Place your fingertips just below your earlobes; gently massage in place using circular motions. Now, slowly move this motion along the jawline toward your chin until your jaw relaxes. Continue this motion for at least a minute.

6. **Cheekbones:** With both hands making a "peace sign," place your index finger just above your upper lip and your middle finger just below your bottom lip. Apply gentle pressure and simultaneously pull your fingers toward your ear. Repeat this action five times.

7. **Scalp:** Make claws with your hands and use your fingertips to rub over your scalp vigorously for two minutes. The pressure force is up to you, but be sure not to use your nails. Instead, use the pads of your fingers. Please pay particular attention to the back of your scalp at the base of your skull, as we carry a lot of tension.

8. **Recover:** Gently place your hands over your eyes and face and inhale deeply through your nose. Exhale slowly through the mouth and repeat until you feel calm.

Face Steaming

Another great way to promote and maintain clear and toned skin (without even touching it) is via steaming. For something so simple, steaming does so much, with Healthline stating that a simple ten-minute steam can provide a whole host of benefits (Santos-Longhurst, 2018).

- **Cleanses the skin.** The heat from steam opens up the pores, loosens any dirt buildup, and prevents sebum (the skin's natural oil) from becoming trapped beneath the surface. This can reduce the chance of breakouts.

- **Promotes circulation.** The warm steam dilates the blood vessels in the face, increasing circulation and producing a natural, healthy glow.

- **Hydrates the skin.** The water droplets of the steam hydrate the skin. The heat also promotes oil production, which naturally moisturizes the face.

- **Improves the absorption of products.** Steam makes the skin more permeable, so you'll get more benefits from skin care products.

- **Promotes collagen and elastin production**. The increased blood flow creates an environment that is great for the production of these substances, resulting in firmer, younger-looking skin.

- **Soothes the mind.** Warm steam on the face is very relaxing. You can even step up the experience and add soothing essential oils to the water for a simultaneous aromatherapy session! BAM!

- **Reduces sinus congestion.** Steams are great to have alongside performing drainage massages, as they relieve sinus congestion by loosening the fluid and mucus that often gets trapped in these areas.

- **Affordable and accessible.** If you have a bowl, a towel, and a way to heat some water, you can enjoy a facial steam.

How to Steam

Fill a bowl with hot water and test the temperature by holding the back of your hand approximately six inches above the water. If this is comfortable for you, sit in front of the bowl and drape a towel over your head and bowl to keep the steam circulating around your face. Stay here for five to ten minutes for all the positive effects to kick in.

Another steaming method is to soak two small towels in a bowl of hot water, wring out the excess, and lightly place them over your face with your nose poking out between them. Lean back in a chair and enjoy!

Poor drainage and circulation are common issues regarding facial rejuvenation, so I recommend trying each technique in this chapter to see which works best for you. Try not to be disappointed if you don't see results immediately. This is the natural method. It can take between two and five weeks to notice a difference. You will experience a more relaxed feeling within your head and facial area before seeing the physical manifestations on the outside. Remember, consistency is key.

Share Your Smile with the World: Be a Hero with Your Review

"The best way to find yourself is to lose yourself in the service of others."

– Mahatma Gandhi

Guess what? People who do kind things for others without waiting for a *"thank you"* often feel happier and more fulfilled. Imagine if we could spread that kind of happiness around! Now, I've got something important to ask you... *Would you be willing to do a small, good deed for someone you've never met?* Even if no one else knew you did it?

Think about it. This person is a lot like you, or maybe like you were once upon a time. They're eager to learn, wanting to make a positive change in their life, and searching for the right guidance but not sure where to turn.

My dream is to make *Facial Fitness: Revolutionize Your Self-care with Facial Exercises and Holistic Massages Techniques for Neck and Décolletage* a tool for everyone. My whole heart is in this mission. To reach this dream, I need to connect with... everyone.

And this is where you, my dear reader, come into play. Believe it or not, many people decide whether to read a book based on what others say about it. So, here's my heartfelt request on behalf of wonderful ladies aged 30-60 who are curious about natural beauty solutions and haven't met you yet:

Please consider leaving a review for this book.

It won't cost you a dime, only a minute of your time, but it could make a world of difference for another person looking to enhance their beauty naturally. Your review might be the key to…

… supporting more small businesses in our communities. …helping another woman provide for her family. …empowering someone to find meaningful work. …assisting another in transforming their life. …making another person's dream a reality.

Feeling that warm, fuzzy feeling inside? That's the joy of helping. And it's super easy to do - just takes a moment to leave a review.

Simply share your thoughts on the website (Amazon, BarnesandNoble, etc.) where you purchased this book.

If you're excited about making a positive impact on someone's journey toward natural and gentle beauty care, then you're exactly who I'm looking for. **Welcome to the family!**

I can't wait to show you how easy it is to reduce signs of aging, boost your skin's health, and find relaxation. The simple tips and natural remedies I've got in store are going to excite and surprise you. A huge thank you from the bottom of my heart. Let's get back to discovering more together.

Your biggest cheerleader, Dr. Andrea Blake-Garrett

P.S. - Here's a little secret: when you share something valuable, you become even more valued. If you know another who would benefit from this book, why not spread the love?

Chapter 6:

Facial Problem Areas

> 66
>
> Don't ask me why I get a massage. Ask yourself why you don't.
>
> **—Unknown**
>
> 99

As you are probably aware, certain areas of the face are considered "problem areas." These areas tend to be the eyes, mouth, and forehead. They are either very stubborn when it comes to improving the signs of aging, or we often neglect or abuse these areas in our day-to-day lives. For example, with the excessive use of technology and screens, our eyes are becoming more dry and thus more puffy-looking. Also, as our sight deteriorates with age, some of us will squint or frown in an attempt to compensate, causing additional creasing or wrinkles on our foreheads. Unfortunately, these actions take their toll on the appearance of our faces, so we should pay extra attention to these areas. This is exactly what the practices in this chapter are going to help you do.

Dominate Tired Eyes

The following practical tips will help you address the dark circles, droopiness, and under-eye puffiness that aging, stress, and unhealthy lifestyle choices, as mentioned earlier, cause.

Use a Compress

Using cool eye pads as soon as you wake up can reduce the puffiness around your eyes throughout the day. As we know, this is because the low temperature helps drain the fluid from this area. Place each one below your bottom lid and keep it in place for at least 10 minutes or as instructed on the packet. Alternatively, cold spoons can be used to gently press down on bags under the eyes until the metal becomes body temperature. Another option is to use green or black tea bags, as the tea contains antioxidants and caffeine, which can constrict blood vessels and reduce inflammation (Silver, 2020). Steep the bags in room temperature water for a few seconds, squeeze out the excess water, and place one under each eye for about 10 minutes.

Sleep With Your Head Raised

Sleep with your head elevated to avoid fluid collecting around your eyes (and face) overnight. Add a few extra pillows so that your upper body is at an angle. If you find this uncomfortable, you could raise one end of the entire bed by driving a wedge under the end where your head lies. There are several types of adjustable beds available online for a long-term solution.

Eye Tapping

1. With clean fingers, gently tap your index and middle fingertips around your eyes for 30 seconds. This will encourage more blood to flow to the area. Continue this tapping action and move out along your eyebrows, down toward your cheekbones, toward the bridge of your nose, and back up to your eyebrows. Circle your eyes like this for 30 seconds.

2. Using the middle finger of each hand, firmly press down on the inner edges of your eyebrows for 10 seconds.

3. With the same fingers, gently press into the sides of your nose by your tear ducts for 10 seconds.

4. Finally, gently massage your temples for 30 seconds.

Eye Pumping (Compression)

1. Gently place your fingertips on the puffy parts under your eyes and perform a light pumping (press and release) action on them for 10 seconds.

2. Move down toward your cheekbones and repeat this action for another 10 seconds.

3. Place your fingertips directly in front of your ears and pump (press and release) for 10 seconds.

4. Repeat this sequence as many times as you feel necessary.

Under-Eye Firming

1. Place your index, middle, and ring fingertips under each eye. They should rest on your cheekbones, approximately a finger width away from your bottom lash line.

2. Gently pull the skins slightly down (this is an exception to the rule) and look up to the ceiling.

3. Slowly blink five times while maintaining the pull with your fingers and looking up.

4. Look diagonally up to the right and repeat another five blinks.

5. Now, look diagonally up to the left and repeat five more blinks.

6. Repeat this sequence for a minute.

Under-Eye Lifting

1. Place the index, middle, and ring fingertips of your right hand on your right cheekbone.

2. Hold the area just below your lower eye lid. Look up and gently pull the skin down. You should feel a slight stretch under your right eye.

3. Use your left-hand fingertips to very gently brush the skin under your right eye up toward your eye in short strokes for 10 seconds. Switch sides and repeat as desired.

Rejuvenate a Lined Mouth and Thin Lips

The mouth and lips are areas that go through a lot as you move through life. Think about all the talking, chewing, and laughing done, not to mention bad habits like smoking or lip-biting. Therefore, I've researched and collected the following tips that will help keep the skin in this area remain smooth, supple, and plump.

Lip Exfoliation

Exfoliating the lips is a great way to introduce some natural color and improve their fullness. The invigoration brings blood to the surface, making them appear more red (a sign of youth), and removing dead skin cells will further enhance this, making them look smoother.

One way to do this is to wet a clean cloth or toothbrush and use it to buff the dead skin away gently. Another option is to create a lip scrub by adding a sprinkle of fine organic brown sugar crystals to your usual lip balm tube. A few drops of peppermint oil or chili powder can also activate the skin. Gently rub this on your lips for a few seconds and wipe away the excess.

Lip Masks

Most of us have heard of face masks, but there are also lip masks that can help tone and moisturize this area specifically. Many store bought face masks avoid the mouth and lips, so these masks are a great way to give some attention to this often neglected area. Lip masks are simple to create yourself using natural ingredients, so why not try one of the following, as recommended by SiO Beauty (Guldager, n.d.)?

- One teaspoon of honey mixed with one teaspoon of lemon juice.

- One teaspoon of yogurt mixed with one half teaspoon of turmeric powder. Use the turmeric sparingly, as it is highly pigmented, and you wouldn't want to be left with yellow lips!

- One teaspoon of olive or castor oil, one half teaspoon of fine brown sugar mixed with a teaspoon of aloe vera gel. Use organic cold-pressed hexane-free castor oil.

Cover your lip with one of these mixtures and leave it on the skin for approximately one to three minutes. When the time is up, gently wash off the mixture with warm water and apply ample lip balm.

Mouth Yoga

1. **Reduce a frowned mouth:** Purse your lips tightly and push them forward as though giving a kiss. Hold this position and

use one hand to place your thumb on one side of the lips and the index finger on the other. Apply some pressure, slowly and firmly drag your fingers away from your lips, smoothing out the skin as you go. Repeat this ten times and relax.

2. **Smooth smile lines:** Relax your mouth and use your index and middle fingers to rub along your smile lines—the lines that run from your nose to the corners of your mouth—for 30 seconds. This will relax these tense muscles and improve blood flow. Next, tap along the line for another 30 seconds.

3. **Smooth upper-lip wrinkles:** Using your thumbs and index fingers, hold both of your lips in a pinch grip. Gently pull your grip forward and outward to stretch your lips. Hold here for five seconds and relax. Repeat five times.

4. **Internal massage:** Close your mouth and use your tongue to massage the inside of your lips and cheeks for 20 seconds. This exercise is often forgotten.

Smooth a Wrinkled Forehead

If you frown a lot or have very expressive eyebrows, the chances are you have more pronounced lines or wrinkles on your forehead than others. These wrinkles aren't necessarily due to age. How you use your frontalis muscle in your face, forehead, and scalp is responsible for these lines. Great news is that, in most cases, those lines are reversible. Therefore, the following tips can help train your forehead and eyebrow muscles to behave in ways that prevent or reduce folds in this area.

Wear Sunglass/Glasses

This is the most simple tip of them all. Wear sunglasses when it's very bright outside, and prescription glasses when needed will prevent you from squinting or frowning unnecessarily. They should also fit well to prevent you from scrunching your nose up to stop them from slipping.

Be Wise With Your Eyes

As you look up and to the sides, many of us will raise our eyebrows unknowingly, thus creating folds in the forehead. This is an unnecessary muscle movement, as it is possible to widen the eyes and look around without using the frontalis muscle. To look up, you only need to use your eye muscles. This is the only movement to aim for. Be wise with your eyes and use those eye muscles only.

To find out how much you use your forehead muscles, place your palm on the area and open your eyes as wide as possible. I can almost guarantee that (unless you've had Botox) your forehead moved considerably. Now, let's try again, but avoid moving your forehead this time. This may be difficult at first, but the more you practice, the lower your chances of creating or worsening lines. Perform this eye-widening exercise 15 times daily, and you'll slowly train your muscles to work for you in this "anti-aging" role.

Frown Line Reduction

1. Using your index fingers, rapidly stroke the area between your eyebrows in an upward motion for 20 seconds. Ensure

that the strokes are short, moderately firm, and only go in one direction.

2. Gradually make the strokes slower and longer until they approach the hairline. Continue for another 20 seconds.

3. Place your index fingers horizontally across the middle of your forehead and apply moderate pressure.

4. While maintaining pressure, pull your fingers apart to gently stretch the skin apart with rapid movements for 20 seconds.

5. Pinch the skin between your eyebrows with your thumb and index finger and, gently pull apart and relax in an outward pumping motion for 20 seconds.

Relax Your Forehead

1. Use your non-dominant hand to hold the top of your forehead in place with your fingertips from above.

2. With the index and middle fingers of the other hand, create continuous firm circles all over the forehead for 30 seconds. Ensure that your face remains relaxed throughout this time.

3. Close your eyes and lightly tap on your forehead for 30 seconds. This should feel very relaxing, like raindrops pattering on your head.

Scar Improvement

If you have any scars on your face or neck from injury or even surgery, I understand this can be difficult to come to terms with. The wounds may have altered your face in undesirable ways, reducing your confidence and sense of self. Fortunately, there are ways to smooth their texture and reduce the tension of the surrounding skin for a more natural look and feel.

Scar Massage

Five-minute daily massages will help scar tissue move freely in all directions, reducing discomfort or pulling. As scar tissue is more rigid than normal skin, it can take up to two years to notice a visual difference, but you may be able to feel the difference in just three weeks of consistent practice.

1. Apply a water-based cream to the scar and massage using your fingertips. Aloe vera gel or creams/oils with high vitamin E content also work well. Be sure to address the skin at least two centimeters around the scar and move in all directions. Continue this for two minutes.

2. Once you feel the scar loosen, you may be able to lift it slightly (if it is small) and roll it between your fingers for another two minutes.

3. Continue to soothe the area by applying a layer of moisturizer every few hours throughout the day.

These "problem areas" can significantly improve without invasive treatment or chemicals. Just be patient, treat your body well from the inside out, and in a few weeks, you will start to notice a difference in even the most stubborn of lines.

Chapter 7:

Neck and Décolletage

> **"**
>
> Aging is a fact of life.
> Looking your age does not
> have to be.
>
> **—Anon**
>
> **"**

The neck and décolletage are two prominent areas where aging can be most pronounced. This is because the skin in this area is notably thinner than in other areas of the body. It may appear to become looser after every birthday. Many people tighten up this area through massage as soon as they notice it heading south.

Neck Massages

Experiencing "turkey neck" is enough to make us fearful of getting older! It's not the most attractive look, but it is very common because the neck is often neglected when it comes to skincare. Excess fat also tends to gather here, making the neck lose its shape and form making you look older. However, plenty of neck and throat massages can be performed to help slow this process down, each with more benefits than you may think!

Recommended oil(s): Natural cold-pressed oils rich in vitamins E and C, such as Jojoba and Sweet almond seed, can help tighten the skin.

Optional tool(s): No tools are necessary for these massages.

Benefits of Neck and Throat Massages

As well as tightening up the skin for a more youthful appearance, there are several other benefits of performing self-massage on the neck and throat.

These massages can:

- Improve the flexibility of the neck. You may have developed some stiffness if you have worked at a desk for years. Fortunately, this can be remedied through massage and stretches.

- Increase the production of endorphins. Endorphins are hormones that make us feel more positive and can boost our self-esteem.

- Strengthen the immune system. Massaging the neck in a particular way will assist with the lymphatic drainage system, thus removing toxins from the body more efficiently.

Another less obvious benefit of neck massage is that it has the potential to improve the voice by manipulating the larynx. This is known as laryngeal massage.

One of the worst-kept secrets about aging is that our muscles become weaker and less defined as we age. According to the UT Southwestern Medical Center, the muscles in our throats are no exception. Yes, our voice box (larynx), vocal cord, and voice-producing mechanisms age with us, and this can cause age-related voice changes (Aging Voice, n.d.). These muscles and surrounding tissues essentially shrink, thin, and stiffen, which can make the voice sound weaker and, in extreme cases, could even cause a slight tremor. Of course, this doesn't happen to everyone, but if you are concerned, you should speak to a medical professional.

Signs of vocal aging include:

- A higher pitch than usual in men.

- A lower pitch than usual in women.

- Loss of projection and resonance. You may find that you can't shout as loudly or clearly as you once could or find yourself squeaking at times.

- Reduced volume and endurance. For example, your normal speaking voice may become quieter and trail off at the end of long sentences.

- Voice tremors (shakiness).

- Weak or breathy voice. It may feel like it's an effort to speak and be heard.

Fortunately, the massages in this chapter will address this internal muscular aging and so much more, leaving you looking (and potentially sounding) more controlled, resonant, and youthful for longer.

Neck Massage Tips

- Start by warming up the neck muscles. This can be done by slowly tilting your head from side to side, looking left and right, and allowing your head to fall back and forward several times.

- Don't forget to take deep, controlled breaths. It is natural to want to hold your breath when working on the primary airway, but this can make you feel dizzy and unintentionally strain your muscles.

- Myofascial release is a technique that helps loosen the tough membranes around your muscles. This can make the skin look smooth and help you feel less tense. The actions best for this area are small circles, elongated passes, and light, sustained pressure.

- When adding oils to the skin of the décolletage, use gentle patting motions (instead of rubbing) if your skin may be particularly sensitive in this area.

Massage 1 – Lifting the Neck

- While looking forward, place the flats of your fingers at the back of your neck, just under your hairline.

- With a firm pressure, start making small circles that slightly pull the skin back and up toward the skull. Keep this going for 30 seconds.

- Staying at the back of the neck, place palm flat against this area. Firmly grab and squeeze (massage) the skin here repeatedly for 30 seconds. Use both hands alternately for even coverage.

- Place the flats of your fingers in the middle of your chest and gently sweep your hand up the center of your neck, out to the right of the jaw, and then down the outer side of your neck. This both lifts the skin and drains the excess fluid from the neck. Alternate sides with each hand for 30 seconds.

- Next, place both thumbs under your chin. Starting close to your neck, apply pressure and drag your thumbs forward while maintaining contact. Repeat ten times.

- Use your index fingers to sweep back and forth across the groove between your chin and bottom lip. It would help if you used your neck muscles to resist this dragging motion and continue for 30 seconds.

- Finally, use the back of your hands to sweep between the chin and neck toward your ears. Alternate sides for 30 seconds to ensure balanced coverage.

Massage 2 – Lengthening the Neck

- Tilt your head to the right and look to the left. You should feel what is known as the sternocleidomastoid (SCM) muscle protrude on the right side of the neck. Gently pinch this muscle with your thumb and hooked index finger to massage it for 10 seconds.

- Repeat this action on the left side for another 10 seconds.

- Using rapid motions, use the backs of your hands to gently pull the skin on the front of your neck back for 30 seconds. Ensure that you cover both sides from top to bottom.

Massage 3 – Myofascial Release

1. Use your thumb and index finger to make small circles along the sides of your larynx (voice box) for 30 seconds.

2. Using the same finger and thumb, start at the top of the throat and slowly glide your fingers down both sides of the larynx until you reach your collarbone. When you reach the bottom of your throat, return to the top and repeat this pass ten times.

3. Now, use both thumbs to gently push up into the soft area under the chin with steady pressure. Hold here for thirty seconds.

4. Next, sit or stand up straight while looking forward. While keeping your shoulders facing forward, turn your head to look to your right and slightly down, as if looking into a pocket on the front of your shirt. You should feel a stretch on the opposite side of the neck. Hold this position and gently glide your hand along the stretched side for up to two minutes.

5. Finally, complete the same stretch on the left.

Lymphatic Drainage (Neck)

There are several lymph nodes around the front, back, and sides of the neck. So, although we have addressed some drainage techniques for the face in Chapter 5, we'll now explore some neck-focused massages that will help remove puffiness from both the face and neck. Do not perform drainage massages if you have an ear, throat, or sinus infection. Unlike working on the face, when draining from the neck, you'll want to work downward toward the collarbone, as this is where the nodes are.

Recommended oil(s): organic base oil such as sunflower, coconut, or jojoba mixed with citrus essential oils.

Optional tool(s): No tools are necessary for this area.

Neck Lymphatic Drainage Tips

- Breathe deeply before starting the massage. Six to ten deep breaths. This wakes up the lymphatic system and acts like a pump, helping the fluid to get moving.

- Use your fingertips to apply controlled, moderate pressure.

- It might be easier to cross your hands when applying pressure to the neck. For example, use your right hand to massage the left side of the neck and the left hand for the right side.

Massage 1 – Surface Movement

1. Stand or sit with your back straight and place both hands at the bottom of your rib cage. Inhale slowly and deeply, as though filling the abdomen with air. Gently sigh as you release the breath out through your mouth. Rest briefly between each breath and repeat five times.

2. Place each hand's index and middle fingers on either side of your neck, just below the earlobes. While applying moderate pressure, gently slide the fingers down toward the shoulders to stretch the skin and release. Repeat this action five times, starting at the earlobes each time.

3. Move your starting position around the jaw and repeat until you have performed steps 5–7 around the whole neck.

4. For the back of the neck, place the flats of your fingers at your nape near the hairline. Apply firm pressure and gently slide the hands down the neck and spine toward the back of the shoulders. Repeat five times, starting at the hairline on the back of the neck each time.

Massage 2 – Full Upper-Body Drainage

This more intense drainage massage will continue draining fluid from the neck to other lymph nodes.

1. Place both hands flat on your stomach. Take a deep breath through your nose until your abdomen extends. Hold for a few moments. Slowly exhale through pursed lips like you are blowing out candles, and let your abdomen return to normal. Repeat this slow breathing five times.

2. Place the flats of your index and middle fingers on either side of your neck and press lightly. While maintaining pressure, massage down and inward along your collarbone without going past it. This should gently stretch the skin of your neck/collarbone and not cause any pain. Release the skin and repeat Steps 5 and 6 10 times. Continue with deep, clearing breaths.

3. Now, place your left palm on your right collarbone and gently pull the skin (not the muscles) down toward your right armpit. To increase the stretch slightly, turn your head to the

left. Repeat this action on the right side of the body another five times.

4. Position your right palm on your left collarbone and gently pull the skin (not the muscles) down toward your right armpit. To increase the stretch slightly, turn your head to the right. Repeat this action on the left side of the body another five times.

5. Place the palm of your left hand against your right armpit. Your fingers should lay in the pit of your arm. Gently pull the armpit up and in toward your body, pause here for a moment, then release. Your hand should be opening and closing your hand each time. Repeat this circular pumping action ten times.

6. Use the right hand to complete the same pumping on your left armpit ten times. Pause in this position for a moment and then release. Repeat five times.

7. Finally, place your hands flat on the back sides of your neck and gently stretch the skin back and down toward your shoulders. Hold here, then release and repeat five times.

As you will be getting a lot of fluid moving during these massages, drinking a glass of water or hydrating juice like pure watermelon or organic coconut water is recommended to help with flushing.

Laryngeal Massage

If you were to go for a spa massage, you would unlikely see "laryngeal massage" on the treatment list. This is because it is a very specialized massage that tends to be saved for speech therapy. It is also challenging to perform on others safely because it is in a vulnerable place, namely because of the sensitivity of the carotid arteries that run down the sides of the neck. You can, however, perform an elementary and more subtle version of this massage on yourself to help improve your vocal strength and tone.

Recommended oil(s): No oils are necessary for this massage, but if you want to benefit from aromatherapy at the same time, you could opt for organic jasmine or lavender. Jasmine oil is believed to resonate with the throat chakra, and lavender relaxes the muscles.

Optional tool(s): No tools are required for this area, as it can be pretty sensitive. A vibrating device can loosen deeper muscles as you become more confident.

Laryngeal Massage Tips

- Warm up your hands before starting so it's easier for your muscles to relax.

- Before starting, have a warm drink to relax the inside of the throat, as well.

- Continue breathing normally while manipulating the area.

Massage 1 – Voice Improvement

1. **SCM massage:** Face forward and use the sides of your index and middle fingers to run down the sides of your neck. Start at your ear and continuously move to the bottom of your neck with moderate pressure for one minute. This massages

the sternocleidomastoid (SCM), the large muscles that run from the middle of the chest to the jaw.

2. **Neck and chin stretch:** Place your hands on your chest to keep the skin in place and tilt your head back—you should feel a mild stretch. While keeping your hands on your chest, briefly stick out your chin and jaw toward the ceiling for a more profound stretch experience in the neck and chin area, then relax. Repeat this "stretch and relax" movement 20 times.

3. **Larynx manipulation:** Face forward and hold the larynx with your thumb and fingers. This might be difficult, but be gentle and patient on your first try. Gently wobble the larynx from side to side for 10 seconds. You might hear a slight click—this is normal—but it shouldn't hurt.

4. **Tongue root:** Place your thumbs under your chin, where you can imagine your tongue root is, and press firmly for 30 seconds.

5. **Jaw release 1:** Press each hand's index and middle fingers on either side of your jaw. Glide your fingers toward your cheekbones and then to your temples while maintaining pressure. Repeat this ten times.

6. **Jaw release 2:** Using your fingertips, find the pocket underneath your cheekbone and press here relatively firmly as you open and close your mouth ten times.

7. **Jaw release 3:** Press your fingers on the sides of your jaw near your earlobes and bite firmly. You should feel some muscles contract. Now, place two fingers on the muscles you felt and gently press into them as your jaw relaxes. Hold here for 20 seconds.

The Impact of Massage on the Thyroid

The thyroid is a gland at the front of the neck that secretes the hormones thyroxine (T4) and triiodothyronine (T3). These hormones help the cells in our bodies perform normally and can affect our metabolism, energy, and mood. Unfortunately, thyroid disorders—when the thyroid secretes too much or too little T3 or T4—are prevalent, especially in women, but massaging this area has been found to benefit those with such disorders in profound ways (Gialelis, 2016). It has the power to reduce symptoms such as thinning hair, dry skin, fatigue, and a puffy face. So, if this is something of a concern for you, massaging the front of the neck may be particularly beneficial.

However, knowing how much or how few hormones will be secreted during a thyroid massage is impossible, so it should not be used to self-medicate. Massage should not replace any medication you are on and should not be performed solely for medical reasons. The main focus of neck massages is to improve aesthetics; any medical improvements are considered a bonus.

Some success stories of thyroid massage have been used to rejuvenate the skin. For example, Aglaia Esthetics Training found that massaging this gland can reduce inflammation in the entire body, improve circulation, and reduce stress, which, as we know, can all have positive effects on the skin (*Aglaia Esthetics Training,* 2019).

Neck Workouts

To achieve longer-lasting results when preventing aging skin around the neck area, it's essential to work the muscles, not just manipulate them. Our muscles begin to deteriorate and weaken without regular stimulation, known as atrophy. This can lead to sagging skin and the buildup of excess fat, so the following workouts are designed to work almost all the muscles in the neck to prevent this from happening. Each can be performed daily and should take less than three minutes to complete.

Option 1

1. **Look left and right:** With your head in a neutral position, slightly draw your chin back (not down) as though trying to give yourself a double chin. Don't worry, this is just temporary! While maintaining this chin position, look to your right, hold for a few seconds, and then look to your left. Repeat this movement ten times.

2. **Head circles:** Bring your head back (not all the way back) to the center and begin making five slow and gentle head circles in a clockwise direction. Change directions, and complete another five circles.

3. **Side to side:** Now, look forward and try to move your head from side to side while keeping your shoulders neutral and chin parallel to the floor. You should always remain looking

forward and only use your neck muscles to move your head. This isn't an easy move, so start slowly and only perform small movements until you are more confident. Repeat ten times.

4. **Chin squares:** Imagine you have a pencil strapped to your chin, pointing down toward the floor. From a neutral position, while keeping your shoulders neutral, move your chin to the left, forward, right, and back, as if drawing a square with the pencil. Continue "drawing" for 30 seconds and repeat the movement in the other direction: right, forward, left, and back. Again, this movement may be tricky, but it will get easier with practice.

5. **Neck flexion:** Stand up straight with your arms resting by your side. Pull your shoulders back and then down while putting your head down and drawing your chin toward your chest. Hold this position for 30 seconds. You should feel a stretch at the back of the neck and potentially between the shoulder blades. If not, you can deepen this stretch by interlocking your fingers and gently pulling down on your head with your hands.

6. **Downward smile:** Lower the corners of your mouth as if making the sound "eeee." Exaggerate this movement as much as possible until tension is created in the neck. Relax and repeat this ten times.

Option 2

1. **Forehead push:** Face forward and stack both hands on your forehead. Use your neck muscles to push your head against your hands, but offer resistance so that your head doesn't move forward. Hold this resistance for 10 seconds, and then relax.

2. **Backward push:** Put your hands behind your head and interlock your fingers. Now push your head backward with your neck muscles but maintain resistance with your hands, and hold for 10 seconds.

3. **Chew:** Sit or stand with your back straight and tilt your head back so your chin is lifted toward the ceiling. With your mouth closed, make an exaggerated chewing motion for 20 seconds.

4. **Kiss:** Like the "chew" exercise, sit or stand with your back straight and tilt your head back. Now, pout 20 times as though blowing a kiss to the ceiling.

5. **Neck lift:** Lie on a bed or a comfortable, safe, raised surface with your head hanging over the edge. If the surface is hard, put some light padding under your neck, but ensure that your head can still hang freely. Slowly lift your head as high as possible, using only your neck muscles, then slowly lower it back down to the starting position. Repeat this five times.

There are plenty of different exercises here to choose from. So, if you find one that is particularly challenging, or causing any discomfort, feel free to mix and match the movements to create a workout plan that works best for you. These exercises shouldn't feel like a chore or burden but part of a positive routine.

Décolletage Massage

The word décolletage comes from a French verb that means "expose the neck." Some consider it one of the most attractive parts of a woman's body, and for men, it is the beginning of the much-desired tight pecs. So, if you've been dreaming of wearing a shirt with a daring, plunging neckline at your next event, décolletage massages will help you show it off in style.

Benefits of Décolletage Massages

The skin on your décolletage area is constantly being pulled and squashed as you move your arms, shoulders, neck, and back. It, therefore, needs a little bit of TLC from time to time to keep the muscles relaxed and smooth. Massage is a great way to do this; it will align the fibers and supply the area with plenty of blood to restore its health.

Did you know there are also such things as "sleep wrinkles?" According to Good Housekeeping, those who sleep on their side can develop fine wrinkles on their chest (Good Housekeeping, 2015). Unfortunately, this can lead to premature sagging, so try to begin your nights on your back if you can. If this is uncomfortable or not possible due to mobility or health reasons, décolletage massage can help smooth them out or even prevent them from happening in the first place.

Recommended oil(s): Organic Jojoba, Aragan, Rose Hip, or Sunflower oil can be used to improve skin elasticity and firmness. It can also plump fine lines and wrinkles when used regularly. You could also add a light exfoliant to the oil, such as brown sugar, to give the area a smooth appearance once the massage is complete.

Optional tool(s): As the skin is delicate in this area, I recommend avoiding the use of tools. Your hand is the best tool to use.

Décolletage Massage Tips

- Perform this massage once a week along with your facial routine.

- You can use this massage as an opportunity to benefit from aromatherapy and use scented oils that will calm or invigorate you for the rest of the day/night.

Massage 1 – Gentle Pressure

1. Warm a few drops of oil in your hands by rubbing them together.

2. Using alternating hands, sweep over the décolletage from one shoulder to the other with medium pressure. Repeat ten times.

3. Gently tilt your head back, then, starting in the middle of the décolletage, sweep your hands up toward the neck with alternating hands. Keep this movement going as you work your way from the left side of the neck to the right for 30 seconds.

4. Place the flats of your fingers in the middle of your chest and press lightly. While maintaining pressure, make small circles as you move across the décolletage towards the right shoulder. When you reach the shoulder, release pressure, return to the center, and start again at the center. Do this five times and then repeat on the left side.

5. Repeat step 2 for 30 seconds, and then place your hands flat on your décolletage to gently calm the skin.

Massage 2 – Rapid Movements

1. Using your left hand, sweep from the back of your right shoulder to the front of your chest ten times. Repeat this on the left shoulder using your right hand.

2. Next, find the depression above your collarbones and use your fingertips to press down into this area with gentle pressure. Move your fingers around until you have covered the entire length of your collarbones.

3. Use the flats of your fingers to rapidly brush from the center of your décolletage toward the shoulder for 30 seconds.

4. Ball your hand into a fist and make small, pressurized circles around the area with the flat part of your knuckles for 30 seconds. Use your left hand for the right side. Your right hand for the left side.

5. Repeat Step 3 to flatten out the muscles again. You are massaging the area under the collarbone. Start near the armpit and move inward to middle of the chest.

Feel free to perform these massages while moisturizing and protecting these often-forgotten body parts with SPF. They will help keep your age a secret for a bit longer and be a novel way to improve your posture as you become prouder to show your neck and décolletage areas off with confidence.

Chapter 8:

On the Chin

> I have what I like to call a "chinneck." My chin just flows rather easily into my neck.
>
> **–Matthew Perry**

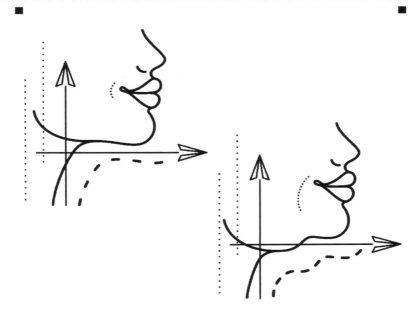

Some people naturally have a less defined jawline, and not much can be done to change this. What most people do have the power to change, however, is the appearance of "jowls" or a "double chin."

Jowls refer to the loose pockets of skin that tend to sag from the chin or jawline just under the corners of the mouth as we age. Almost everyone gets them to varying degrees. Their severity usually involves genetics and environmental or lifestyle choices, such as regular facial expressions, weight loss, and posture. Once they develop, they are difficult to reduce without surgery or expensive procedures, so it is ideal to prevent them from developing in the first place.

A double chin is the collection of fat or loose skin that hangs under the chin, giving the appearance of two chins. Weight gain is the most common reason for getting them. However, gravity, time, and age can be factors. Unfortunately, our increased use of cell phones and technology that require a bowed head is also to blame as the weight of our head presses down on the throat, creating folds. So, staying on top of your health and skincare is vital to slow this process down.

Chin Massages

If you have a full beard, you probably won't notice some of the effects of aging on the chin so much—lucky you! However, if you still want to try a rejuvenating massage, I recommend only attempting massages 1 and 3, as massage 2 (gua sha) may be difficult/impossible to execute correctly. If you have a low beard or stubble, feel free to use all methods, as the skin and hair follicles underneath the hair will benefit from additional blood flow.

Recommended oil(s): Olive and almond oils are great for tightening the skin due to their high levels of vitamin E. Shea butter, or argan oil is excellent for reducing itching and frizz if you have facial hair. Organic oils are best.

Optional tool(s): A gua sha can be used for these massages, as its groove is perfect for getting into the angles of the chin. Gua Shas are nor very expensive. It is your choice whether to use it or your hands.

Chin Massage Tips

- As with our face massages, you should massage the chin upward to go against gravity.

- After your massage, try sleeping on a high pillow that elevates your chin. This helps reduce the chances of developing a double chin by keeping your head and neck in a neutral position.

- If you have facial hair, try to be gentle and ensure that your movements go toward the hair growth. Constantly manipulating "against the grain" can be uncomfortable and may cause excess pulling, skin trauma, and hair loss.

Massage 1 – No Tools

1. **Chin pulls:** Use your thumb and index finger to hold your chin. While maintaining this grip, move your fingers along your jawline towards your ear. Repeat ten times. You can also perform the "pull" along the jawline using the palm of your hand.

2. **Jaw pinches:** Create a hook shape with your index fingers and place them at the front of your chin. Keep them there and put your thumbs just below your earlobes. Now, drag your index fingers toward your thumbs along your jawline until you gently pinch the skin by your ears. Hold here for a few moments and release. Repeat this ten times.

3. **Knuckle glides:** Bend your index fingers and place the flat part of your knuckles on the front of your chin. Gently glide them both out toward your ears and repeat ten times.

4. **Jaw brushes:** Use your left hand's index and middle fingers to hold the skin below your bottom lip. Then, with the same

two fingers of your right hand, use small, rapid strokes to brush up toward your cheeks from the jawline. Move along the entire right side of the jaw, then repeat on the left for 20 seconds.

5. **Cheek pinch:** With your index fingers and thumbs in pincer-like positions, place both of your index fingers on your right cheek and both of your thumbs just under your chin. Slowly bring your thumbs up toward your finger and allow it to glide along the skin. Gently pinch the gathered skin for a few moments and repeat ten times, ensuring you cover the entire right side of the face. Repeat on the left side.

6. **Chin hold:** Rest your elbows on a chest-height surface and place your hands by your face. Relax your face into your hands, allowing gravity to pull your head down slightly. You should feel light tension in the skin under your chin. Hold here for 30 seconds, rest, and repeat.

Massage 2 – Gua Sha

1. **Outward stroke:** Using the most extended and flattest side of your gua sha, gently place it where your neck meets the back of your chin and drag the tool forward ten times. You are always starting at the back of the chin.

2. **Chin/jaw stroke:** Place your left thumb under the tip of your chin to hold the skin in place. Hold the gua sha with your right hand and gently use it to pull the skin from where your thumb is back toward the neck, and then up toward the right

ear. Hold here for a few seconds, repeat this movement ten times, and switch sides, remembering to always work in one direction.

3. **Jaw Definition:** Use your fingertips to press down on the skin just under your bottom lip. Place your jaw between the groove on the M-shaped side of the gua sha and slowly move the tool from your fingers to the right ear.

4. **Cheek Hold:** Place the side of your left hand on the right side of the nose and mouth and apply light pressure to keep the skin in pace. Using the long, flat side of your gua sha gently glide it across the cheek from your hand to the ear ten times. Repeat on the left side of the face.

Massage 3 – Facial Hair Treatment

If you have a beard or mustache, the following massage will be easier to follow while addressing the skin beneath. Although facial hair can disguise many signs of aging or bad habits, the chin and mouth areas shouldn't be neglected entirely, as you could end up with clogged pores and a dull complexion. Massage in this area can eliminate "beardruff" (dandruff of the beard), decrease itchiness, and prevent ingrown hairs. Some believe it may even make the hair grow faster and slow the appearance of grays due to improved blood circulation if this is something you desire (Bhowmik, 2022)!

1. **Prepare the Hair:** Dampen your beard with warm water, then apply your chosen oil to your hands and rub them together to warm/loosen it up. Gently rub the oils into your

beard and mustache hair and, if long enough, detangle them with a wide-toothed comb.

2. **Beard Stretch:** Using long strokes, glide the palms of your hands from the ears down along the jawline and toward your chin. Continue this motion to the end of your beard. Repeat this five times.

3. **Improve Circulation:** Gently pull the skin under your beard with rapid pinching from the right ear, along the jaw, and to the left ear. Go back and forth with this motion for 30 seconds.

4. **Exfoliate:** Lift your chin and claw your hands. Use your fingertips to softly scratch under the chin toward the neck rapidly for 30 seconds. Be sure to cover all areas of the chin and beard.

5. **Chin Awakening:** Place the length of your right index finger in the groove between your bottom lip and chin and apply slight pressure. Swipe the finger out to the right and repeat ten times. Switch fingers and then repeat toward the left.

6. **Soothe the Skin:** Warm your hands by rubbing them together for 30 seconds. Apply your hands to your chin and hold here for another 30 seconds. Feel free to use a warm cotton rag/towel instead of hands.

Chin and Neck Yoga

Yoga is an ancient physical and spiritual practice that aligns the energies of the mind, body, and soul. It was first developed in India and has been used for over 5,000 years to promote flexibility, endurance, strength, calmness, and well-being in people of all ages, backgrounds, and walks of life (Nichols, 2021). In fact, it is so popular that one in seven adults in the United States has tried it (Nichols, 2021)!

Full-body yoga involves getting into positions that help us think and feel positive while using breathing techniques to keep us calm and grounded. Neck and chin yoga is simply an extension of this but only uses the muscles and positions of the head, chin, and neck to achieve similar results. So, use the following moves to not only give you more taut, flexible, and relaxed muscles in this area but will also help you de-stress and enjoy getting to know your skin on a deeper level.

Recommended oil(s): As you won't be touching your chin or neck very much, massage oils are optional. However, before starting, I recommend applying some light moisturizer or oil on the area to avoid cracking the skin as it is stretched.

Optional tool(s): No tools are necessary for these movements. However, a yoga mat will add some comfort when performing the stretches that involve the whole body.

Routine 1 – Combat a Saggy Neck

1. **Ceiling kisses:** From a neutral position, tilt your head up to look at the ceiling. While in this position, make repetitive and

exaggerated kissing faces for 20 seconds. You should feel a slight pull or tightening of chin and middle neck area.

2. **Smile soother:** Use one of your index fingers to press firmly on your chin. Then, tick your lips under your teeth and smile as much as possible. Open and close your mouth with your lips in this position repeatedly while slowly moving your head back and forth. Keep these movements going for 20 seconds.

3. **Swan neck:** From a neutral position, turn your head to the right as if trying to look into the pocket at the back of your pants. Keep your shoulders facing forward and hold here for 10 seconds. Return to neutral and repeat on the left side. Do not tilt your head down.

4. **Neck extension:** Gently place your fingers on your collarbone and stick your lower lip out. While keeping it protruding, slowly tilt your neck back and hold it to a point where you feel a nice deep stretch along the front of your neck. Hold for 10 seconds while breathing slowly and deeply through your nose. Return to neutral and repeat this extension five times.

5. **Pinch and lift:** With your head facing forward, use your fingertips to pinch and lift the skin on your neck gently. Start by your collarbone and work your way up to the jaw. Perform these pinches for 20 seconds.

Routine 2 – Neck Tightening

1. **Pouting Lift:** Stick your lower lip out to make a pouting face and hold it there for a few seconds. With your lip still protruding, open and close your mouth ten times. Rest and repeat for another set.

2. **Chewing Gum:** Turn your head to the right, and while keeping your mouth closed, perform an exaggerated chewing motion for 10 seconds. Pause, turn your head to the left, and repeat.

3. **Swallowing Stretch:** Tilt your head back to look at the ceiling. With your mouth open, touch your tongue to the roof of your mouth and gently swallow. This will be an unusual sensation, so take your time and relax. Swallow four times and rest. Next, turn your head to the right and swallow in the same way for more times. Then, turn to the left and repeat.

4. **Upward-Facing Dog:** This stretch involves the whole body and provides a long, deep stretch along the chin, neck, and chest area. Lie face down on the floor and use your arms to push your upper body up until they are straight. Keep your hips in contact with the floor and look up toward the ceiling. Hold here for 10 seconds, and then relax. Repeat four times.

Routine 3 – Battling a Double Chin

1. **Fish Face:** Firmly suck in your cheeks and hold for 30 seconds while breathing normally through your nose. Relax and then repeat five times.

2. **Lion Pose (Simha mudra):** Kneel on the floor with your back straight and sit on your heels if you can. If this is uncomfortable, sitting on a chair is fine. Rest your hands on your thighs and stick your tongue out as much as possible without straining your muscles. Inhale deeply through your mouth and roaring like a lion as you exhale. Repeat five times.

3. **Tongue Lock (Jivha Bandha):** Sit facing forward and open your mouth. Place your tongue on the roof of your mouth and look at the center of your nose. Slowly inhale, exhale through your mouth, and hold this position for 20 seconds.

4. **Face Purification (Kapal dhouti):** Sit with a straight back and place your fingertips together. Inhale deeply and then hold your breath. Puff your cheeks out and use your thumbs to hold your nostrils closed. While continuing to hold your breath and nostrils, bow your head so that your chin touches your chest and pause here for 10 seconds or for as long as you can. Slowly exhale through your nose and repeat three times.

Routine 4 – Full Body Poses with Chin and Neck Sculpting Benefits

The following poses involve the whole body, so grab a mat and gently warm up the body by jogging on the spot for a minute. They may be a bit of a challenge for newbies but do your best and enjoy the holistic benefits.

1. **Stick Pose (Chaturanga Dandasana):** Lie face down on your mat with your palms flat at either side of your ribs. Curl your toes under and push your entire body off the floor while remaining flat like you're performing a plank. Hover about six inches over the floor like this for about 10 seconds (or as long as you can) while looking down at your mat. Relax and then repeat five times. This pose requires some good upper-body and core strength, so do your best and work from there.

2. **Dolphin Pose (Ardha Pincha Maryurasana):** Kneel on your mat and place your palms and forearms flat before you. Now, tuck your toes under and inhale as you push up with your legs to make a triangle shape with your body. Keep looking at your hands and breathe normally. Hold here for 10 seconds and then relax. Repeat five times.

3. **Camel Pose (Ustrasana):** Kneel on your mat without sitting on your heels. Arch your back backward as you look up toward the ceiling. If you can, touch your ankles and hold for 10 seconds. Breathe gently through your nose with your mouth closed and relax. Repeat five times.

Chapter 9:

Full Face Workouts

> **"**
>
> Laughter is the sun that drives winter from the human face.
>
> **–Victor Hugo**
>
> **"**

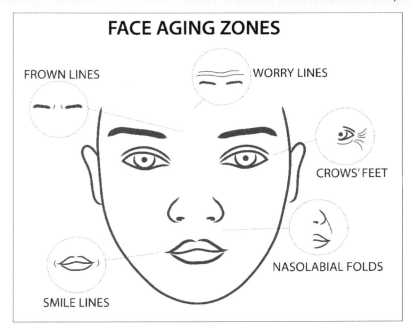

FACE AGING ZONES

FROWN LINES

WORRY LINES

CROWS' FEET

NASOLABIAL FOLDS

SMILE LINES

You should grab a mirror for this chapter; it could be hilarious! It will involve making some unflattering facial expressions, but I promise it will all be worth it. There are 43 muscles in the face. The facial nerve controls most of them.

Facial Workouts

Each of the following exercises will work the muscles of your face in ways that keep "problem areas" taut and other places, like the upper jaw and scalp, tension-free to help you feel relaxed. They can be repeated daily to gradually tone your muscles, slim the face, and energize as you dominate the day ahead.

Facial exercises work as aging remedies because firmer muscles help hold fat pockets in place, reducing the chances of the "droopy" look associated with aging, and it can take as little as three weeks to notice the difference (Collins, n.d). This is all very exciting, but don't rush the process. Always build up intensity gradually, as you can pull a muscle in any part of the body!

Recommended oil(s): No oils are necessary as you won't touch your face too much. However, to avoid stretching or cracking dry skin, ensure that your face and lips are well moisturized.

Optional tool(s): A spoon is required for workout 3.

Facial Workout Tip

- Never overwork the muscles. Despite having so many muscles in your face, you shouldn't feel "the burn" like you would after going to the gym.

- Between workouts, try to perfect good tongue posture. Not many people know this, but your tongue should always be lying flat against the top of your mouth. According to Well & Good, this will help subtly lift the cheekbones and eliminate jowls. It will also open the nasal airways better, an excellent tip for snorers (Rud, 2022).

Workout 1 – Upper Face

1. **Brow raises:** Place each hand's index and middle fingers directly above your eyebrows. Gently push the skin down until your eyelids feel slightly hooded. Using the muscles in your forehead, try lifting your fingers ten times. Rest and then repeat.

2. **Eyelid stretch:** With your eyes open, use the heels of your hands to pull your eyebrows up toward your forehead gently. While holding your eyebrows up, slowly blink ten times. This will help smooth wrinkles around the eyes.

3. **Crows feet:** Squeeze both eyes shut firmly, but not so hard that it becomes uncomfortable. Hold for a second, and then relax. Repeat this squeeze ten times. This will help smooth wrinkles around and on the outer corners of the eyes, also known as "crow's feet."

4. **Eye lift:** With your eyes open, lift your lower lids to meet your upper ones. It should feel as though you are squinting. Repeat this ten times.

5. **Upper face stretch:** Use your index fingers and thumbs to create C shapes and place them around your eyes. Your index fingers should be above your eyebrows, and your thumbs should be below your cheekbones. Shut your eyes and slowly use your hands to squeeze your face inwards, then relax the tension and pull your face outward. Hold here for five seconds, and then repeat another four times.

Workout 2 – Lower Face

1. **Cheek lift:** Place your index and middle fingers on your cheekbones and gently lift the skin until taut. While holding the skin in place, open your mouth as wide as you can comfortably or until you feel resistance in your cheek

muscles. Hold this position for five seconds and repeat five times.

2. **Cheek squeeze:** Tilt your head back and suck your cheeks as much as possible. Hold for five seconds, then release. Repeat this ten times.

3. **Pufferfish:** Close your mouth and gently puff your cheeks out. Move the air from left to right, filling one cheek at a time for 30 seconds. Rest and repeat.

4. **Big smile:** Twenty-six of the forty-three muscles of the face are used for smiling. Place your fingertips on your cheeks and smile widely. While smiling, gently pull your cheeks up and hold for 10 seconds. Relax and then repeat five times. Do several repetitions throughout the day and enjoy looking younger by toning your facial muscles.

5. **Big kiss:** Pout your lips and stick them out as far as possible. Hold here for a second, then pull them back into a closed-mouth smile. Go from a pout to smile relatively quickly, ten times.

6. **Thumb suck:** Place a clean thumb in your mouth and make an exaggerated sucking expression. Hold here for two seconds, and then relax. Repeat ten times.

Workout 3 – Lower Face

1. **Mouth pulse:** Wash your hands and hook your index fingers around the corners of your mouth. Gently pull your mouth apart and then contract the muscles around your mouth to

pull your fingers toward each other in a pulsing motion. Continue this for 15 seconds, pause, and then repeat.

2. **Laughter line pull:** Tuck your lips underneath your teeth and hold them in place with moderate pressure. Next, place your index fingers flat on your laughter lines—either side of your mouth. Apply pressure with your fingers and gently pull them apart, stretching your mouth area. Hold here for 10 seconds and relax. Repeat five times.

3. **Cheek crunches:** Face forward and rest your left hand flat against the side of your face. Hold the skin in place as you blow in short, sharp bursts to the right. Keep your head facing forward, and imagine trying to blow a feather off your right shoulder. Repeat this ten times and then switch sides.

4. **Lip to nose:** Tilt your head back and purse your lips together as though giving a kiss. Use your mouth muscles to pull your top lip up to touch your nose briefly and relax. Repeat this upward motion ten times.

5. **Spoon lift:** Face forward and fold your lips inward. Place the handle tip of a clean spoon between your lips and allow the spoon to drop slightly by relaxing the tension between your lips. Then, quickly tense the mouth muscles to bring the spoon up to 90 degrees/parallel to the floor. Hold here for five seconds, then relax. Repeat this spoon lift five times.

6. **Spoon pull:** Face forward and fold your lips inward. Place the handle between your lips horizontally and hold it in place

for a few seconds. Now, use your hands to gently pull the spoon away from your face, but use your mouth and chin muscles to add resistance. Hold this pull for five seconds and relax. Repeat five times.

Workout 4 – Full Face Routine

1. **OO-EE:** Using exaggerated expressions, make the sounds "OO" and then "EE." When saying "OO" raise your eyebrows simultaneously for an extra workout in the forehead. Go back and forth between the sounds ten times, then relax. Repeat another ten times.

2. **Raspberries:** Just as you did when you were younger, take a deep breath and blow a big, long raspberry with your jaw, cheeks, and lips fully relaxed. Keep blowing raspberries for 30 seconds.

3. **Touch your nose:** Open your mouth wide and stick your tongue out. Now, try to touch the tip of your nose with your tongue five times, then relax. Repeat another round.

4. **Upper-lip pout:** Open your mouth very slightly and relax your jaw. Keep your bottom lip still as you pout with just your top lip. Relax and repeat rapidly 20 times.

5. **Cheek risers:** Start with a neutral expression. Now, try raising your cheeks without smiling. This may involve simultaneously using your lower eyelids, nose, and cheek muscles. Repeat ten times, rest, and repeat.

Yoga for the Face

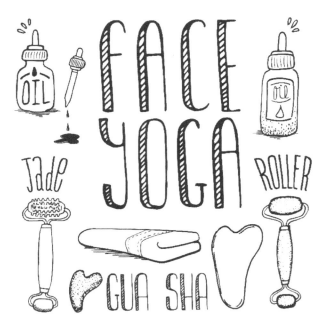

The following yoga routines have been inspired by The Yoga Expert, Danielle Collins, and other notable facial fitness experts. They are each designed to help you look three years younger in just five months using traditional techniques alongside more modern moves with scientifically proven results (Collins, n.d.).

Face Yoga Tips

- Practice face yoga twice daily, once in the morning and once at night. It can take as little as five minutes, so do your best to fit it in for your well-being.

- Complete your routine in front of a mirror because, with face yoga, the aim is not to have any creases or folds in the skin.

- Take your time. You only need to complete three or four exercises per session and change the routine daily.

- Face yoga is more complicated than it looks! As challenging as it is, try not to hold your breath or tense your muscles when unnecessary. It will get easier, so persevere, and you'll be a face yogi in no time.

Optional tool: A pencil, chopstick, or straw can be used in routine 2.

Routine 1 – Improve Definition

1. **Eye and cheek definition**: Reach up and over your head with your left arm and place your fingertips on the right side of your face, by your temple. Put your head down so your left ear moves toward your left shoulder, and hold here for a few seconds. Slowly use your fingertips to gather and gently pull the skin beside your eye toward your eyebrow and take a deep breath. Sharply, breathe out through your mouth with your tongue out. Relax and repeat five times. Now, perform this on the right side five times.

2. **Cheekbone definition:** Place your index and middle fingers under your cheekbones and apply light pressure with your fingertips. Quickly push upward and out from your nose towards your ear. Release the skin from under your fingers in a flicking motion, and repeat rapidly twenty times. Breathe deeply and slowly through your nose as you go. Rest and repeat.

3. **Jaw definition:** Ensure your chin remains parallel to the floor and your neck is straight. Smile widely and use the backs of your fingers to tap under the chin for 30 seconds.

Routine 2 – General Anti-Aging

1. **Eye-opener:** Place your hands around your eyes as if forming a pair of binoculars and apply firm pressure. Attempt to lift your eyebrows while holding this shape and resisting these movements. Relax and then squint. Repeat this lift and squint forty times.

2. **Forehead lifter:** Interlock your fingers and place them on your forehead. Apply a light pressure and lift the skin toward your hairline. Pulse here for one minute.

3. **Cheek lifter:** Cover your teeth with your lips and open your mouth widely. Hold this position for 10 seconds, then return to a neutral position. Repeat this ten times.

4. **Smile lifter:** Sit tall, with your shoulders aligned and neck straight. Put a straw or pencil between your lips and hold it in place with your lips. With the item still between your lips, attempt to smile while keeping it still. You should feel the muscles in your cheeks and around your mouth working. Hold here for 10 seconds, and then relax. Repeat four times.

As suggested in previous chapters, feel free to mix and match the exercises in each routine to find your perfect yoga session. Simply follow the instructions and tips and enjoy the benefits. You look marvelous!

Keeping the Game Alive

Congratulations! You've journeyed through the pages of this book and now hold the secrets to defying aging, melting away stress, enhancing your skin's vitality, expanding your knowledge on self-care, and establishing a beauty routine that fits seamlessly into your life. It's a powerful toolkit you've acquired, and it's time to share the wealth of knowledge you've gained.

Your experience and insights are invaluable, not just to you but to others on a similar quest for health and beauty. By sharing your honest thoughts about this book on Amazon, BarnesandNoble, or wherever you purchased this book, you're lighting the way for more individuals, both women and men aged 30 and up, guiding them towards the transformative power of Facial Fitness Exercises and Massage Techniques.

Here's your chance to pass the torch of wisdom and inspire a passion for facial fitness in others. Your review isn't just feedback; it's a beacon for those seeking guidance and a testament to the impact this book has had on your life.

We're all part of a larger journey toward health and wellness, and your contribution keeps this vibrant community thriving. The legacy of Facial Fitness Exercises and Massage Techniques grows with each person it touches, and by sharing your journey, you're not just recommending a book—you're enriching lives.

As we close this chapter, remember that the journey of self-improvement and discovery never truly ends. By leaving your review, you're not just helping to keep the game alive; you're playing an integral role in a community that values growth, health, and the timeless beauty of knowledge shared.

I am grateful for your help and for joining me in this mission to spread the word about the power of facial fitness. Your review is more than just words; it's a gift that keeps on giving, helping others to find their path to wellness and beauty, just as you have.

Thank you for choosing to be a part of this movement. Your support and willingness to share your journey make all the difference. Together, we're not just embracing self-care; we're revolutionizing it, one review at a time.

With gratitude,

Dr. Andrea Blake-Garrett (Dr. ABG)

Conclusion

> Time spent getting a
> massage is never a waste.
>
> —Anon

Throughout this book, I've demonstrated that we can control the signs of aging, skin and muscle health, and even hormonal issues into our own hands—literally—naturally and cost-effectively. Our face is a massive part of our identity. Improving aspects of what you aren't happy with through massage, exercise, and lifestyle changes is valid for your self-esteem and confidence. One of the most essential things you cannot ignore is nutrition's role in helping one look marvelous at any age. Collagen, for example, is necessary to prevent our skin from sagging. It provides a firmer, more youthful look to the body and face. You want to consume foods rich in protein, Vitamin C, Vitamin A, etc. Vitamin C helps regenerate skin cells and aids in the reduction of wrinkles. Being consistent with your nutritional intake will help you dominate your look.

Remember that facial massages are available to all, and you don't need to indulge in state-of-the-art equipment or expensive gadgets to reap its benefits. Just your hands and favorite organic oils will do the job very well. It's also essential to work from the inside out. A healthier you mentally, emotionally, spiritually, and physically allows you to dominate your goals. Armed with this knowledge, we can always ensure that we look MARVELOUS at any age.

Tailor Your Massage or Workout

Facial Fitness: revolutionize your Self-care with Facial Exercises and Massage Techniques for the Face & Neck and Décolletage covers many different facial massage and workout techniques, each with benefits, from lymphatic drainage to laryngeal massage, stone scraping to facial yoga. I've included the table below to help you create a massage routine addressing your concerns and goals. Refer to it as needed.

	Type of Massage/Workout					
Concern	Drainage	Circulation	Gua Sha	Lifting	Laryngeal/ Throat	Workout/Yoga
Puffiness	X		X		X	
Double chin			X	X		X
Sagging neck			X	X	X	X
Dull complexion	X	X	X			X
Acne	X	X				X
Dry skin		X				

	Type of Massage/Workout					
Concern	Drainage	Circulation	Gua Sha	Lifting	Laryngeal/ Throat	Workout/Yoga
Oily skin	X					X
Sensitive skin	X	X				X
Aging voice					X	
Wrinkles		X		X		X
Excessive tension		X	X			X

Each massage, used with the best oil for your skin, can help you feel like a new person without stepping foot in a doctor's surgical suite. In a few short weeks, you (and your friends) are bound to notice a difference, much like the thousands of people who have benefitted from face fitness across the globe.

As someone who greatly values mental, emotional, spiritual, and physical health and wellness, practicing facial fitness and massage has been exceptionally beneficial to maintaining my 100-pound weight loss transformation. Not only did it reduce my signs of aging, but it also aided in detoxification, boosted circulation, and relieved physical afflictions like headaches and sinus issues. Considering all this, we deserve access to these practical and surprisingly easy techniques. Use them to achieve your dream of looking beautiful or handsome on the outside while feeling energized and confident on the inside, too.

Thank you for trusting the process and joining me on this journey to aging gracefully while learning how to show up as your most authentic self. Whether you are 38, 58, 68, or older, continue this journey toward a rejuvenated, sculpted, more youthful face with pride because YOU ARE WORTH IT! Continue to live fit and free for life. YOU LOOK MARVELOUS!

About the Author

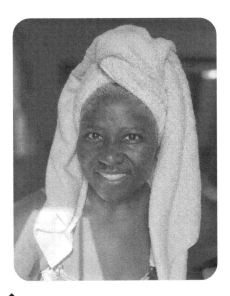

> **"** If I can see the sunshine through
> the rain, I WIN.
>
> **—Dr. Andrea Blake-Garrett, Age 53** **"**

Dr. Andrea Blake-Garrett is a talented author, educator, and entrepreneur known for her education and health and wellness work. She firmly believes that a healthy mind, body, and spirit are the keys to a fulfilling life. Her journey toward transformation began in December 2020, when she decided to take charge of her health and make significant changes in her lifestyle.

Dr. Blake-Garrett lost an incredible 100 pounds of body fat through sheer determination, consistency, and hard work. Her success inspired her to create Teamnoexcuses50, a health and wellness company that helps clients of all ages adopt healthier lifestyles. With her experience and knowledge in health and wellness, Dr. Blake-Garrett has significantly impacted many people's lives.

Dr. Blake-Garrett is also a Cancer Action Network Advocate working continuously with the American Cancer Society and active social media user, with her Instagram handle, the "Notorious Dr. ABG," gaining momentum. She uses her platform to share valuable insights on health and wellness, motivate and inspire her followers, and advocate for a healthier lifestyle for all.

As an author, Dr. Blake-Garrett has published six books. Her fourth book, *DOWN 100 Pounds! How I Used Positive Affirmations To Transform My Mind & Help Maximize My Weight Loss and Life!* documents her journey toward weight loss and offers practical tips for others who want to follow in her footsteps. Her fifth book, *Life! Spice It Up! How To Transform and Heal With 5 Everyday Spices* highlights spices' medicinal properties and how they can be used to promote and maintain better health. The sixth book, *Live Fit & Free For Life: Exercise for Seniors 60+*, outlines the aging process and what happens to the body as you age. It addresses common fears and frustrations often experienced by older adults and provides practical advice on overcoming them.

Overall, Dr. Andrea Blake-Garrett is a passionate and dedicated wife, mom of twins, author, educator, and health and wellness advocate who has made it her mission to help others to "Power Up" lead healthier, happier, and more fulfilling lives. She truly believes anyone can achieve their health and wellness goals with the right mindset and accurate information.

References

Aberin, D. (2022, June 29). *Forty quotes about celebrating your inner beauty.* The Gaggler. https://thegaggler.com/40-powerful-quotes-to-celebrate-your-inner-beauty/

Aging voice. (n.d.). UT Southwestern Medical Center. https://utswmed.org/conditions-treatments/aging-voice/

Aglaia Esthetics Training. (2019, April 1). *How to massage the thyroid gland.* YouTube. https://www.youtube.com/watch?v=HHTbNLvr1g4

The benefits of getting a facial for men. (2021, January 11). Carisma Spa & Wellness. https://www.carismaspa.com/blog-backend/the-benefits-of-getting-a-facial-for-men

Bhowmik, S. (2022, October 18). *Seven things to do everyday to make your beard grow much faster.* MensXP. https://www.mensxp.com/grooming/beards-and-shaving/45267-7-things-to-do-everyday-to-make-your-beard-grow-much-faster.html

Biswas, C. (2021, October 4). *10 neck tightening exercises to get rid of double chin.* StyleCraze. https://www.stylecraze.com/articles/turkey-neck-exercises/

Bowman, J. (2020, July 30). *The four best vitamins for your skin.* Healthline. https://www.healthline.com/health/4-best-vitamins-for-skin

CBC. (2019). *The seven universal emotions we wear on our face.* CBC. https://www.cbc.ca/natureofthings/features/the-seven-universal-emotions-we-wear-on-our-face

CDC. (2019). *Frequently asked questions – Alcohol.* Centers for Disease Control and Prevention. https://www.cdc.gov/alcohol/faqs.htm

Cirino, E. (2017, April 18). *Can you treat turkey neck?* Healthline. https://www.healthline.com/health/beauty-skin-care/turkey-neck#exercises

Collins, D. (n.d.). *Danielle Collins, The face yoga expert.* Face Yoga Expert. Retrieved February 17, 2023, from https://faceyogaexpert.com

Cronkleton, E. (2020, May 12). *Eight benefits of facial massage.* Healthline. https://www.healthline.com/health/beauty-skin-care/facial-massage-benefits#purported-benefits

Cult Fit. (2021, November 8). *Five minute face yoga for double chin.* YouTube. https://www.youtube.com/watch?v=u15R_E60kEI

Curtiss, A. (2018, March 21). *Top seven myths about facials and skincare debunked!* Make Me Fab. https://www.makemefab.com/facials/top-7-myths-about-facials-and-skincare-debunked/

Davids, L. (2020, July 9). *Gua Sha massage: The history, benefits, and side effects.* The Skin Games. https://www.theskingames.com/gua-sha-the-history-benefits-and-side-effects/

Davison, E. (2023, January 27). *This is the correct order to apply your skincare products.* Cosmopolitan. https://www.cosmopolitan.com/uk/beauty-hair/a29263234/correct-order-to-apply-skincare-products/

DeSantis, L. (2018, March 20). *Is acupressure the secret to a glowing complexion?* Health. https://www.health.com/beauty/acupressure-glowing-skin

Fifty massage quotes. (n.d.). Ambient Noise. https://ambientnoise.online/50-massage-quotes/

Florida Academy. (2019, May 17). *The history of massage therapy: 5,000 years of relaxation and pain relief.* Florida Academy. https://florida-academy.edu/history-of-massage-therapy/

Gialelis, J. (2016, January 6). *Massage therapy & thyroid health.* Massage Magazine. https://www.massagemag.com/massage-therapy-thyroid-health-34099/

Gillette. (2019, July 24). *How to stop oily skin: A man's guide.* Gillette. https://www.gillette.co.uk/blog/how-to-shave/a-mans-guide-to-oily-skin/

Good Housekeeping. (2015, November 3). *Nine reasons to start caring for your décolletage.* Good Housekeeping. https://www.goodhousekeeping.com/uk/fashion/a557796/9 -reasons-caring-for-your-decolletage/

Guldager, A. (n.d.). *12 easy tips for soft, smooth, kissable Lips.* SiO Beauty. Retrieved February 16, 2023, from https://www.siobeauty.com/blogs/resource-center/how-to- get-soft-lips

Hallberg, J. (2020, March 19). *Forty-one spa & massage therapy quotes (pampering & relaxation).* The Salon Business. https://thesalonbusiness.com/spa-quotes/

Harper, L. (2023, January 30). *Would you want a stranger's fingers in your mouth? I find out why celebrities love buccal massage.* The Guardian. https://www.theguardian.com/fashion/2023/jan/30/why- celebrities-love-buccal-massage-mouth-facial

Health and Well-being. (n.d.). *Pressing too hard at temple.* Similar Worlds. Retrieved February 18, 2023, from https://similarworlds.com/health-well-being/4327103- Pressing-too-hard-at-temple-My-chiropractor-is

The history of massage therapy. (2018, August 27). WellSpring School of Allied Health. https://wellspring.edu/massage- therapy/history-massage-therapy/

Jacob, D. (2021, May 6). *How much collagen should you take a day?* MedicineNet.

https://www.medicinenet.com/how_much_collagen_should
_you_take_a_day/article.htm

Jahns, E. (2022, July 27). *Coconut oil: What's the verdict on using it for skin? We settle the debate.* Byrdie. https://www.byrdie.com/coconut-oil-for-skin

Johnson, C. (2017, May 10). *Suffering from vocal tension? Give yourself a massage!* The Naked Vocalist. https://www.thenakedvocalist.com/vocal-tension-self-massage/

Johnson, J. (2020, October 30). *Jawzrsize review: Does it work?* Medical News Today. https://www.medicalnewstoday.com/articles/jawzrsize-review

Klasovsky, L. (2020, November 30). *A simple nine-step DIY facial massage for glowing skin.* Mind Body Green Lifestyle. https://www.mindbodygreen.com/articles/diy-facial-massage-for-glowing-skin

Kobido—the best face massage ever. (2021, March 1). The L.A. Glow. https://thelaglow.com/kobido/

Kolli, G. (2022, March 20). *Six facial yoga techniques to reduce your double chin.* Solara Home. https://www.solara.in/blogs/home-fitness/facial-yoga-techniques-to-reduce-your-double-chin

Kubala, J. (2022, August 17). *Do you need supplements for better skin? Here's what science says.* Healthline.

https://www.healthline.com/health/beauty-skin-care/supplements-for-better-skin

La Forge, T. (2021, December 10). *How to use herbs for anxiety and stress.* Healthline. https://www.healthline.com/health/mental-health/herbs-for-stress-recipe

La Sante. (2014, May 30). *Indian head massage—history, treatments and benefits. La Sante.* https://www.lasante.com.au/indian-head-massage-history-treatments-and-benefits/

Levy, J. (2022, July 15). *Seven face yoga exercises to try now.* Dr. Axe. https://draxe.com/beauty/face-yoga-exercises/

Lien-Lun Chien, A. (n.d.). *Sunscreen and your morning routine.* Hopkins Medicine. https://www.hopkinsmedicine.org/health/wellness-and-prevention/sunscreen-and-your-morning-routine

LIHA. (2021, December 19). Skin-to-skin: *What African traditions teach us about facial massage and self care.* LIHA Beauty. https://lihabeauty.com/blogs/journal/skin-to-skin-what-african-traditions-teach-us-about-facial-massage-and-self-car

L'Oréal Paris. (n.d.). *The Jacquet massage technique... Someone pinch me, please.* L'Oréal Paris. Retrieved February 7, 2023, from https://www.lorealparis.co.in/the-jacquet-massage-technique-someone-pinch-me-please

Ludwig, J. (2020, July 6). *Beyond coconut: Seven other natural oils for smooth and radiant skin.* Everyday Health. https://www.everydayhealth.com/skin-and-beauty/best-natural-oils-healthy-skin/

Massage Works. (2017, June 7). *The history of massage therapy.* Massage Works Therapy Center. https://www.massageworksfw.com/blog/the-history-of-massage-therapy/

Mirabello, S. (2019, February 21). *How can gut health affect your skin.* Now Patient. https://nowpatient.com/blog/healthy-living-and-wellness/how-can-gut-health-affect-your-skin-and-why

Myofascial release techniques & stretches for the throat. (n.d.). University of Mississippi Medical Center. Retrieved February 10, 2023, from https://www.umc.edu/Healthcare/ENT/Patient-Handouts/Adult/Speech-Language-Pathology/Voice/Circumlaryngeal-Massage.html

Nakin Skincare. (2020, June 11). *Natural alternatives to synthetic peptides in skin products.* Nakin Skincare. https://www.nakinskincare.com/blogs/news/natural-alternatives-to-synthetic-peptides-in-skin-products

Natale, N., & Smith, J. (2021, November 17). *Thirty-five celebrities on the best parts of aging.* Prevention.

https://www.prevention.com/health/g27558841/age-quotes/?slide=15

Natural Body. (n.d.). *Five essential oils to use in massage.* Natural Body Spa and Shop. https://www.naturalbody.com/blog/5-essential-oils-to-use-in-massage

Nichols, H. (2021, April 15). *How does yoga work?* Medical News Today. https://www.medicalnewstoday.com/articles/286745

Perkins, S. (2021, February 12). *Weird, but normal, body reactions of aging.* Mayo Clinic Health System. https://www.mayoclinichealthsystem.org/hometown-health/speaking-of-health/weird-but-normal-body-reactions-of-aging

Poidevin-Hill, S. (n.d.). *How a five minute "at home" facial massage can help reduce anxious thoughts and facial tension.* Wǒ. https://wearewo.com/blogs/journal/how-a-five-minute-at-home-facial-massage-can-help-reduce-anxious-thoughts-and-facial-tension

Robert A. *Heinlein quotes.* (n.d.). Brainy Quote. https://www.brainyquote.com/quotes/robert_a_heinlein_12 1947

Rud, M. (2022, November 2). *I tried this 3-minute face sculpting workout every day for a week, and actually noticed a difference.* Well+Good. https://www.wellandgood.com/face-workout/

Santos-Longhurst, A. (2018, July 10). *10 benefits of face-steaming and how to do it at home.* Healthline; Healthline Media. https://www.healthline.com/health/benefits-of-steaming-face

Seven herbal alternatives to cosmetics. (2013, June 10). The Health Site. https://www.thehealthsite.com/beauty/herbal-alternatives-to-cosmetics-61044/

Shah, M. (2020, August 5). *10 things people can do to maintain their youth.* American Society of Plastic Surgeons. https://www.plasticsurgery.org/news/blog/ten-things-people-can-do-to-maintain-their-youth

Silver, N. (2020, June 30). *10 ways to get rid of puffy eyes.* Healthline. https://www.healthline.com/health/eye-health/how-to-get-rid-of-puffy-eyes

Slater, D. (2020, March 23). *The history of massage therapy.* Keheren Therapy. https://www.keherentherapy.co.uk/history-massage-therapy/

Step-by-step natural facial massage. (n.d.). Center of Excellence. Retrieved February 18, 2023, from https://www.centreofexcellence.com/natural-facial-massage-guide/

Swedish Massage - The Complete Guide. (2018, February 25).
American Institute of Clinical Massage.
https://www.aicm.edu/blog/2018/2/25/swedish-massage-
expect

Tabner, C. (2022, February 14). *How to massage scars and scar
tissue.* My Expert Midwife.
https://myexpertmidwife.com/blogs/my-expert-
midwife/how-to-massage-scars-and-scar-tissue

Taktak, A. (2022, July 2). *Face, neck, and back muscles:
Anatomy and overview.* Study.com.
https://study.com/learn/lesson/face-neck-muscles-
anatomy-
overview.html#:~:text=These%2520muscles%2520act%2520
to%2520raise

Times of India. (2020, April 15). *Five facial yoga tips to get rid of
your double chin.* The Times of India.
https://timesofindia.indiatimes.com/life-style/health-
fitness/weight-loss/5-facial-yoga-tips-to-get-rid-of-your-
double-chin/photostory/75143436.cms

Valenti, L. (2015, January 21). *What's that like? 10 celebrities
with the world's most perfect skin.* Marie Claire Magazine.
https://www.marieclaire.com/beauty/news/g2610/celebritie
s-with-amazing-skin/

Veurink, E. (2022, December 10). *I tried it: A week of daily facial massages*. Byrdie. https://www.byrdie.com/facial-massage-5187961

Villines, Z. (2022, July 29). *Anti-aging face massage: Benefits and how to try*. Medical News Today. https://www.medicalnewstoday.com/articles/anti-aging-face-massage#does-it-work

Wallersteiner, R. (2021, January 11). *Reflexology: What is it and what are the health benefits?* Netdoctor. https://www.netdoctor.co.uk/healthy-living/a3055/health-benefits-of-reflexology/

White, T., Milliken, L., & A Fisher, M. (2021, August 11). *Empowering healthy eating in America*. Federation of American Scientists. https://fas.org/blogs/sciencepolicy/empowering-healthy-eating-in-america/

Yaminah Abdur-Rahim. (2018, October). *Everything you need to know about facial cupping*. Healthline; Healthline Media. https://www.healthline.com/health/facial-cupping

Image References

Afonshina, Mariana. "Jade Facial Massage"
https://www.shutterstock.com/image-vector/jade-facial-
massage-woman-face-lines-2013922574. Accessed 12 January
2024.

Bagrina, Alla. "Face Aging Zones"
https://www.shutterstock.com/image-vector/womans-face-
places-where-wrinkles-appear-499866715. Accessed 12 January
2024.

Blake-Garrett, Andrea. Selfie Headshot. 3 October 2023, Personal
Collection of Dr. Andrea Blake-Garrett, New Jersey.

Epana. "Yoga For Face" https://www.shutterstock.com/image-
vector/set-gua-sha-massage-tools-facial-1701476497. Accessed
12 January 2024.

Lena, Pani. "Chinneck – Double Chin"
https://www.shutterstock.com/image-vector/double-chin-icon-
set-outlines-half-1677177103. Accessed 12 January 2024.

Michinoku. "Facial Mask Sheet"
https://www.shutterstock.com/image-vector/instruction-how-
apply-facial-sheet-mask-652499875. Accessed 12 January 2024.

Nadiinko. "Skin care Line Icon Set"
https://www.shutterstock.com/image-vector/skin-care-line-icons-set-moisture-2274164057. Accessed 12 January 2024.

ORLY Designs. "Facial Muscles of the Female"
https://www.shutterstock.com/image-vector/facial-muscles-female-detailed-bright-anatomy-1964154679. Accessed 12 January 2024.

ORLY Designs. "Woman Face Superficial Deep Muscle Scheme"
https://www.shutterstock.com/image-vector/woman-face-superficial-deep-muscles-scheme-2329463041. Accessed 12 January 2024.

Zubada. "Female Portrait with Lymphatic Massage Scheme"
https://www.shutterstock.com/image-vector/female-portrait-lymphatic-massage-scheme-1571332798. Accessed 12 January 2024.

Made in the USA
Columbia, SC
25 September 2024

43006757R00100